KT-592-669

Immunology at a Glance

J.H.L. Playfair

Emeritus Professor of Immunology
University College London Medical School
London

B.M. Chain

Professor of Immunology
University College London Medical School
London

Tenth Edition

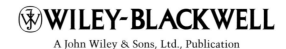
WILEY-BLACKWELL
A John Wiley & Sons, Ltd., Publication

This edition first published 2013
© 2013 by John Wiley & Sons, Ltd.
Previous editions: 1979, 1982, 1984, 1987, 1992, 1996, 2001, 2005, 2009

Wiley-Blackwell is an imprint of John Wiley & Sons, formed by the merger of Wiley's global
Scientific, Technical and Medical business with Blackwell Publishing.

Registered office: John Wiley & Sons, Ltd, The Atrium, Southern Gate, Chichester, West Sussex,
PO19 8SQ, UK

Editorial offices: 9600 Garsington Road, Oxford, OX4 2DQ, UK
The Atrium, Southern Gate, Chichester, West Sussex, PO19 8SQ, UK
111 River Street, Hoboken, NJ 07030-5774, USA

For details of our global editorial offices, for customer services and for information about how to
apply for permission to reuse the copyright material in this book please see our website at www.
wiley.com/wiley-blackwell.

The right of the authors to be identified as the authors of this work has been asserted in accordance
with the UK Copyright, Designs and Patents Act 1988.

All rights reserved. No part of this publication may be reproduced, stored in a retrieval system, or
transmitted, in any form or by any means, electronic, mechanical, photocopying, recording or
otherwise, except as permitted by the UK Copyright, Designs and Patents Act 1988, without the
prior permission of the publisher.

Designations used by companies to distinguish their products are often claimed as trademarks. All
brand names and product names used in this book are trade names, service marks, trademarks or
registered trademarks of their respective owners. The publisher is not associated with any product or
vendor mentioned in this book. This publication is designed to provide accurate and authoritative
information in regard to the subject matter covered. It is sold on the understanding that the publisher
is not engaged in rendering professional services. If professional advice or other expert assistance is
required, the services of a competent professional should be sought.

Library of Congress Cataloging-in-Publication Data
Playfair, J. H. L.
Immunology at a glance / J.H.L. Playfair, B.M. Chain. – 10th ed.
p. ; cm. – (At a glance series)
Includes bibliographical references and index.
ISBN 978-0-470-67303-4 (pbk. : alk. paper) – ISBN 978-1-118-44745-1 (eBook/ePDF) –
ISBN 978-1-118-44746-8 (ePub) – ISBN 978-1-118-44747-5 (eMobi)
I. Chain, B. M.   II. Title.   III. Series: At a glance series (Oxford, England)
[DNLM: 1. Immune System Phenomena. QW 540]

616.07'9–dc23

2012024675

A catalogue record for this book is available from the British Library.

Wiley also publishes its books in a variety of electronic formats. Some content that appears in print
may not be available in electronic books.

Cover image: courtesy of Science Photo Library
Cover design by Meaden Creative

Set in 9/11.5pt Times by Toppan Best-set Premedia Limited, Hong Kong
Printed and bound in Malaysia by Vivar Printing Sdn Bhd

1   2013

Immunology at a Glance

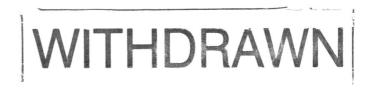

LIVERPOOL JMU LIBRARY

3 1111 01406 9189

Companion website

This book has a companion website at:

www.ataglanceseries.com/immunology

The website includes:
- 95 interactive test questions
- All figures from the book as PowerPoints for downloading

Contents

Companion website

This book has a companion website at:

www.ataglanceseries.com/immunology

The website includes:
- 95 interactive test questions
- All figures from the book as PowerPoints for downloading

Preface

This is not a textbook for immunologists, who already have plenty of excellent volumes to choose from. Rather, it is aimed at all those on whose work immunology impinges but who may hitherto have lacked the time to keep abreast of a subject that can sometimes seem impossibly fast-moving and intricate.

Yet everyone with a background in medicine or the biological sciences is already familiar with a good deal of the basic knowledge required to understand immunological processes, often needing no more than a few quick blackboard sketches to see roughly how they work. This is a book of such sketches, which have proved useful over the years, recollected (and artistically touched up) in tranquillity.

The Chinese sage who remarked that one picture was worth a thousand words was certainly not an immunology teacher, or his estimate would not have been so low! In this book the text has been pruned to the minimum necessary for understanding the figures, omitting almost all historical and technical details, which can be found in the larger textbooks listed on the next page. In trying to steer a middle course between absolute clarity and absolute up to dateness, we are well aware of having missed both by a comfortable margin. But even in immunology, what is brand new does not always turn out to be right, while the idea that any form of presentation, however unorthodox, will make simple what other authors have already shown to be complex can only be, in Dr Johnson's heartfelt words, 'the dream of a philosopher doomed to wake a lexicographer'. Our object has merely been to convince workers in neighbouring fields that modern immunology is not quite as forbidding as they may have thought.

It is perhaps the price of specialization that some important aspects of nature lie between disciplines and are consequently ignored for many years (transplant rejection is a good example). It follows that scientists are wise to keep an eye on each others' areas so that in due course the appropriate new disciplines can emerge – as immunology itself did from the shared interests of bacteriologists, haematologists, chemists and the rest.

J.H.L. Playfair
B.M. Chain

Acknowledgements

Our largest debt is obviously to the immunologists who made the discoveries this book is based on; if we had credited them all by name it would no longer have been a slim volume! In addition we are grateful to our colleagues at UCL for advice and criticism since the first edition, particularly Professor J. Brostoff, Dr A. Cooke, Dr P. Delves, Dr V. Eisen, Professor F.C. Hay, Professor D.R. Katz, Dr T. Lund, Professor P.M. Lydyard, Dr D. Male, Dr S. Marshall-Clarke, Professor N.A. Mitchison and Professor I.M. Roitt. The original draft was shown to Professor H.E.M. Kay, Professor C.A. Mims and Professor L. Wolpert, all of whom made valuable suggestions. We would like to thank Dr Mohammed Ibrahim (King's College Hospital), Dr Mahdad Noursadeghi (UCL) and Dr Liz Lightsone (Imperial College) for help with the new chapters in the ninth edition. Edward Playfair supplied a useful undergraduate view of the first edition. Finally, we would like to thank the publishing staff at Wiley-Blackwell for help and encouragement at all stages.

Note on the tenth edition

Since the last edition in 2009 every chapter has needed some updating, but the major advances concern the innate immune system, whose cells, molecules and receptors continue to attract enormous attention from immunologists. We have added a new chapter on cytokine receptors, and completely rewritten the chapter on autoimmunity. Some chapters have been moved to fit better into the sequence of a typical undergraduate course – for example AIDS and evolution, and the clinical section has been expanded to include a brief survey of methods in use in the immunology lab. Self-assessment now includes online MCQs as well as the essay-type questions at the end of the book.

J.H.L. Playfair
B.M. Chain

How to use this book

Each of the figures (listed in the contents) represents a particular topic, corresponding roughly to a 45-minute lecture. Newcomers to the subject may like first to read through the **text** (left-hand pages), using the figures only as a guide; this can be done at a sitting.

Once the general outline has been grasped, it is probably better to concentrate on the **figures** one at a time. Some of them are quite complicated and can certainly not be taken in 'at a glance', but will need to be worked through with the help of the **legends** (right-hand pages), consulting the **index** for further information on individual details; once this has been done carefully they should subsequently require little more than a cursory look to refresh the memory.

It will be evident that the figures are highly diagrammatic and not to scale; indeed the scale often changes several times within one figure. For an idea of the actual sizes of some of the cells and molecules mentioned, refer to **Appendix I**.

The reader will also notice that examples are drawn sometimes from the mouse, in which useful animal so much fundamental immunology has been worked out, and sometimes from the human, which is after all the one that matters to most people. Luckily the two species are, from the immunologist's viewpoint, remarkably similar.

Further reading

Abbas AK, Lichtman AH, Pillai S. (2011) *Cellular and Molecular Immunology*, 7th edn. Elsevier, Saunders (560 pp.)

DeFranco AL, Locksley RM, Robertson M. (2007) *Immunity*. Oxford University Press, Oxford (350 pp.)

Delves PJ, Martin S, Burton DR, Roitt IM. (2011) *Roitt's Essential Immunology*, 12th edn. Wiley-Blackwell, Oxford (560 pp.)

Gena R, Notarangelo L. (2011) *Case Studies in Immunology: A Clinical Companion*, 6th edn. Garland Science Publishing, New York (376 pp.)

Goering RV, Dockrell HM, Zuckerman M, Roitt IM, Chiodini PL (2012) *Mims' Medical Microbiology*, 5th edn. Elsevier, London

Kindt TJ, Osborne BA, Goldsby R. (2006) *Kuby Immunology*, 6th edn. W.H. Freeman, New York (603 pp.)

Murphy K. (2012) *Janeway's Immunobiology*, 8th edn. Garland Science Publishing, New York (868 pp.)

Playfair JHL, Bancroft GJ. (2012) *Infection and Immunity*, 4th edn. Oxford University Press, Oxford (375 pp.)

List of abbreviations

ACTH	adenocorticotrophic hormone		GH	growth hormone
ADA	adenosine deaminase		GM	granulocyte–monocyte
ADCC	antibody-mediated cellular cytotoxicity		GM-CSF	granulocyte macrophage colony-stimulating factor
ADH	antidiuretic hormone		GMP	guanosine monophosphate
AIDS	acquired immune deficiency syndrome		GVH	graft-versus-host
ALS	antilymphocyte antisera		GVT	graft-versus-tumour
AMP	adenosine monophosphate		HAART	highly active antiretroviral therapy
ANA	antinuclear antibody		HBV	hepatitis B virus
APC	antigen-presenting cell		HDL	high-density lipoprotein
ARC	AIDS-related complex		HEV	high endothelial venule
ARDS	adult respiratory distress syndrome		HHV	human herpes virus
β2M	β_2-microglobulin		HIV	human immunodeficiency virus
BALT	bronchial-associated lymphoid tissue		HLA	human leucocyte antigen
BCG	bacille Calmette–Guérin		HPV	human papillomavirus
BSE	bovine spongiform encephalopathy		HS	haemopoietic stem cell
CAH	congenital adrenal hyperplasia		HTLV	human T-cell leukaemia virus
cAMP	cyclic AMP		ICAM	intercellular adhesion molecule
CCL	chemokine ligand		IDC	interdigitating dendritic cell
CCR	chemokine receptor		IFN	interferon
CEA	carcinoembryonic antigen		Ig	immunoglobulin
CFU-GEMM	colony-forming unit – granulocyte, erythroid, monocyte, megakaryocyte		IL	interleukin
			ITAM	immunoreceptor tyrosine-based activation motif
CGD	chronic granulomatous disease		ITIM	immunoreceptor tyrosine-based inhibitory motif
cGMP	cyclic GMP		JAK	Janus kinase
CJD	Creutzfeldt–Jakob disease		KIR	killer inhibitory receptor
CK	cytokine		KSHV	Kaposi sarcoma-associated herpes virus
CLV	central longitudinal vein		LC	Langerhans' cell
CMI	cell-mediated immunity		LH	luteinizing hormone
CMV	cytomegalovirus		LPS	lipopolysaccharide
CON A	concanavalin A		LRR	leucine-rich repeat
CR	complement receptor		LS	lymphoid stem cell
CREST	calcinosis, Raynaud's, oesophageal dysmotility, sclerodactyly, telangiectasia (syndrome)		LT	leukotriene
			MAC	macrophage
CRP	C-reactive protein		MAF	macrophage activating factor
CSF	cerebrospinal fluid		MALT	mucosa-associated lymphoid tissue
CSF	colony-stimulating factor		MBL	mannose-binding lectin
CTL	cytotoxic T lymphocyte		MBP	mannose-binding protein
DAF	decay accelerating factor		M-CSF	macrophage colony-stimulating factor
DAMP	damage-associated molecular pattern		MHC	major histocompatibility complex
DC	dendritic cell		MIF	macrophage migration inhibition factor
DSCG	disodium cromoglicate		MK	megakaryocyte
DTH	delayed-type hypersensitivity		MMR	measles, mumps and rubella
EBV	Epstein–Barr virus		MPS	mononuclear phagocytic system
EL	efferent lymphatic		MRSA	methicillin-resistant *Staphyloccus aureus*
ELISA	enzyme-linked immunosorbent assay		MW	molecular weight
ER	endoplasmic reticulum		NBT	nitroblue tetrazolium (test)
ES	erythroid cell		NK	natural killer
FACS	fluorescence-activated cell sorting		NO	nitric oxide
FDC	follicular dendritic cell		PAMP	pathogen-associated molecular pattern
FSH	follicle-stimulating hormone		PC	plasma cell
G6PD	glucose-6-phosphate dehydrogenase		PCD	programmed cell death
GALT	gut-associated lymphoid tissue		PCR	polymerase chain reaction
GBM	glomerular basement membrane		PCV	post-capillary venule
G-CSF	granulocyte colony-stimulating factor		PG	peptidoglycan

PG	prostaglandin		**SNP**	single nucleotide substitution
PGL	progressive generalized lymphadenopathy		**SOD**	superoxide dismutase
PHA	phytohaemagglutinin		**SSPE**	subacute sclerosing panencephalitis
PK	pyruvate kinase		**STAT**	signal transducer and activator of transcription
PL	prolactin		**TAA**	tumour-associated antigen
PMN	polymorphonuclear leucocyte		**TAP**	transporter of antigen peptide
PNP	purine nucleoside phosphorylase		**TB**	tuberculosis
PRR	pattern-recognition receptor		**TCGF**	T-cell growth factor
RA	rheumatoid arthritis		**TCR**	T-cell receptor
RAG	recombination activating gene		**TD**	thoracic duct
RER	rough endoplasmic reticulum		**TGF**	transforming growth factor
RES	reticuloendothelial system		**TIL**	tumour-infiltrating lymphocyte
RF	rheumatoid factor		**TLR**	Toll-like receptor
Rh	Rhesus		**TNF**	tumour necrosis factor
ROS	reactive oxygen species		**TRH**	TSH-releasing hormone
SALT	skin-associated lymphoid tissue		**TSH**	thyroid-stimulating hormone
SIV	simian immunodeficiency virus		**VCAM**	vascular cell adhesion molecule
SLE	systemic lupus erythematosus			

1 The scope of immunology

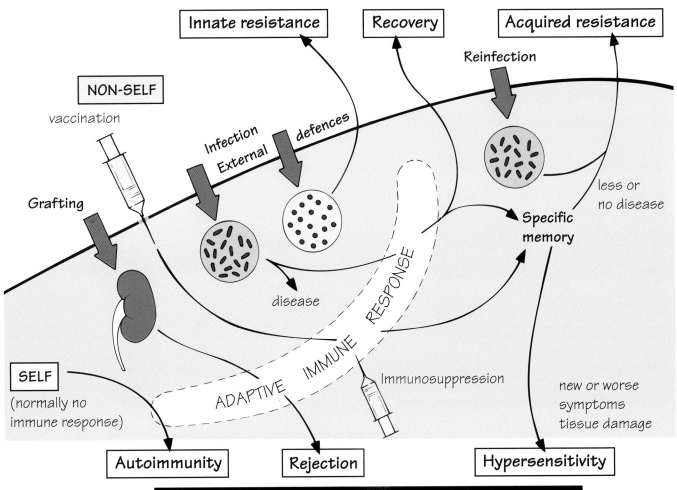

Of the four major causes of death – injury, infection, degenerative disease and cancer – only the first two regularly kill their victims before child-bearing age, which means that they are a potential source of lost genes. Therefore any mechanism that reduces their effects has tremendous survival value, and we see this in the processes of, respectively, **healing** and **immunity**.

Immunity is concerned with the recognition and disposal of foreign or 'non-self' material that enters the body (represented by red arrows in the figure), usually in the form of life-threatening infectious microorganisms but sometimes, unfortunately, in the shape of a life-saving kidney graft. Resistance to infection may be '**innate**' (i.e. inborn and unchanging) or '**acquired**' as the result of an **adaptive immune response** (centre).

Immunology is the study of the organs, cells and molecules responsible for this recognition and disposal (the 'immune system'), of how they respond and interact, of the consequences – desirable (top) or otherwise (bottom) – of their activity, and of the ways in which they can be advantageously increased or reduced.

By far the most important type of foreign material that needs to be recognized and disposed of is the microorganisms capable of causing infectious disease and, strictly speaking, immunity begins at the point when they enter the body. But it must be remembered that the first line of defence is to keep them out, and a variety of **external defences** have evolved for this purpose. Whether these are part of the immune system is a purely semantic question, but an immunologist is certainly expected to know about them.

 Immunology at a Glance, Tenth Edition. J.H.L. Playfair and B.M. Chain. © 2013 John Wiley & Sons, Ltd. Published 2013 by John Wiley & Sons, Ltd.

Non-self A widely used term in immunology, covering everything that is detectably different from an animal's own constituents. Infectious microorganisms, together with cells, organs or other materials from another animal, are the most important non-self substances from an immunological viewpoint, but drugs and even normal foods, which are, of course, non-self too, can sometimes give rise to immunity. Detection of non-self material is carried out by a range of **receptor** molecules (see Figs 5, 10–14).

Infection Parasitic viruses, bacteria, protozoa, worms or fungi that attempt to gain access to the body or its surfaces are probably the chief *raison d'être* of the immune system. Higher animals whose immune system is damaged or deficient frequently succumb to infections that normal animals overcome.

External defences The presence of intact skin on the outside and mucous membranes lining the hollow viscera is in itself a powerful barrier against entry of potentially infectious organisms. In addition, there are numerous antimicrobial (mainly antibacterial) secretions in the skin and mucous surfaces; these include lysozyme (also found in tears), lactoferrin, defensins and peroxidases. More specialized defences include the extreme acidity of the stomach (about pH 2), the mucus and upwardly beating cilia of the bronchial tree, and specialized surfactant proteins that recognize and clump bacteria that reach the lung alveoli. Successful microorganisms usually have cunning ways of breaching or evading these defences.

Innate resistance Organisms that enter the body (shown in the figure as dots or rods) are often eliminated within minutes or hours by inborn, ever-present mechanisms, while others (the rods in the figure) can avoid this and survive, and may cause disease unless they are dealt with by adaptive immunity (see below). These mechanisms have evolved to dispose of pathogens (e.g. bacteria, viruses) that if unchecked can cause disease. Harmless microorganisms are usually ignored by the innate immune system. Innate immunity also has a vital role in initiating the adaptive immune response.

Adaptive immune response The development or augmentation of defence mechanisms in response to a particular ('specific') stimulus, e.g. an infectious organism. It can result in elimination of the microorganism and recovery from disease, and often leaves the host with specific memory, enabling it to respond more effectively on reinfection with the same microorganism, a condition called acquired resistance. Because the process by which the body puts together the receptors of the adaptive immune system is random (see Fig. 10), adaptive immunity sometimes responds to harmless foreign material such as the relatively inoffensive pollens, etc., or even to 'self' tissues leading to **autoimmunity**.

Vaccination A method of stimulating the adaptive immune response and generating memory and acquired resistance without suffering the full effects of the disease. The name comes from vaccinia, or cowpox, used by Jenner to protect against smallpox.

Grafting Cells or organs from another individual usually survive innate resistance mechanisms but are attacked by the adaptive immune response, leading to rejection.

Autoimmunity The body's own ('self') cells and molecules do not normally stimulate its adaptive immune responses because of a variety of special mechanisms that ensure a state of self-tolerance, but in certain circumstances they do stimulate a response and the body's own structures are attacked as if they were foreign, a condition called autoimmunity or autoimmune disease.

Hypersensitivity Sometimes the result of specific memory is that re-exposure to the same stimulus, as well as or instead of eliminating the stimulus, has unpleasant or damaging effects on the body's own tissues. This is called hypersensitivity; examples are allergies such as hay fever and some forms of kidney disease.

Immunosuppression Autoimmunity, hypersensitivity and, above all, graft rejection sometimes necessitate the suppression of adaptive immune responses by drugs or other means.

2 Innate and adaptive immune mechanisms

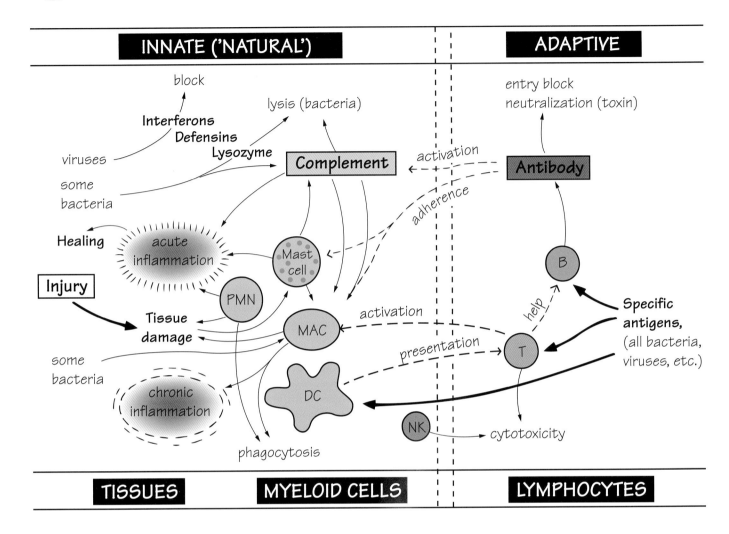

Just as resistance to disease can be innate (inborn) or acquired, the mechanisms mediating it can be correspondingly divided into **innate** (left) and **adaptive** (right), each composed of both **cellular** (lower half) and **humoral** elements (i.e. free in serum or body fluids; upper half). Adaptive mechanisms, more recently evolved, perform many of their functions by interacting with the older innate ones.

Innate immunity is activated when cells use specialized sets of receptors (see Fig. 5) to recognize different types of microorganisms (bacteria, viruses, etc.) that have managed to penetrate the host. Binding to these receptors activates a limited number of basic microbial disposal mechanisms, such as phagocytosis of bacteria by macrophages and neutrophils, or the release of antiviral interferons. Many of the mechanisms involved in innate immunity are largely the same as those responsible for non-specifically reacting to tissue damage, with the production of **inflammation** (cover up the right-hand part of the figure to appreciate this). However, as the nature of the innate immune response depends on the type of infection, the term 'non-

specific', although often used as a synonym for 'innate', is not completely accurate.

Adaptive immunity is based on the special properties of **lymphocytes** (T and B, lower right), which can respond selectively to thousands of different non-self materials, or '**antigens**', leading to specific memory and a permanently altered pattern of response – an *adaptation* to the animal's own surroundings. Adaptive mechanisms can function on their own against certain antigens (cover up the left-hand part of the figure), but the majority of their effects are exerted by means of the interaction of antibody with complement and the phagocytic cells of innate immunity, and of T cells with macrophages (broken lines). Through their activation of these innate mechanisms, adaptive responses frequently provoke **inflammation**, either acute or chronic; when it becomes a nuisance this is called **hypersensitivity**.

The individual elements of this highly simplified scheme are illustrated in more detail in the remainder of this book.

Innate immunity

Interferons A family of proteins produced rapidly by many cells in response to virus infection, which block the replication of virus in the infected cell and its neighbours. Interferons also have an important role in communication between immune cells (see Figs 23 and 24).

Defensins Antimicrobial peptides, particularly important in the early protection of the lungs and digestive tract against bacteria.

Lysozyme (muramidase) An enzyme secreted by macrophages that attacks the cell wall of some bacteria.

Complement A group of proteins present in serum which when activated produce widespread inflammatory effects, as well as lysis of bacteria, etc. Some bacteria activate complement directly, while others only do so with the help of antibody (see Fig. 6).

Lysis Irreversible leakage of cell contents following membrane damage. In the case of a bacterium this would be fatal to the microbe.

Mast cell A large tissue cell that releases inflammatory mediators when damaged, and also under the influence of antibody. By increasing vascular permeability, inflammation allows complement and cells to enter the tissues from the blood (for further details of this process see Fig. 7).

PMN Polymorphonuclear leucocyte (80% of white cells in human blood), a short-lived 'scavenger' blood cell whose granules contain powerful bactericidal enzymes. The name derives from the peculiar shapes of the nuclei.

MAC Macrophage, a large tissue cell responsible for removing damaged tissue, cells, bacteria, etc. Both PMNs and macrophages come from the bone marrow, and are therefore classed as **myeloid** cells.

DC Dendritic cells present antigen to T cells, and thus initiate all T-cell-dependent immune responses. Not to be confused with follicular dendritic cells, which store antigen for B cells (see Fig. 19).

Phagocytosis ('cell eating') Engulfment of a particle by a cell. Macrophages and PMNs (which used to be called 'microphages') are the most important phagocytic cells. The great majority of foreign materials entering the tissues are ultimately disposed of by this mechanism.

Cytotoxicity Macrophages can kill some targets (perhaps including tumour cells) without phagocytosing them, and there are a variety of other cells with cytotoxic abilities.

NK (natural killer) cell A lymphocyte-like cell capable of killing some targets, notably virus-infected cells and tumour cells, but without the receptor or the fine specificity characteristic of true lymphocytes.

Adaptive immunity

Antigen Strictly speaking, a substance that stimulates the production of **antibody**. However, the term is applied to substances that stimulate any type of adaptive immune response. Typically, antigens are foreign ('non-self') and either particulate (e.g. cells, bacteria) or large protein or polysaccharide molecules. Under special conditions small molecules and even 'self' components can become antigenic (see Figs 18–21).

Specific; specificity Terms used to denote the production of an immune response more or less selective for the stimulus, such as a lymphocyte that responds to, or an antibody that 'fits' a particular antigen. For example, antibody against measles virus will not bind to mumps virus: it is 'specific' for measles.

Lymphocyte A small cell found in blood, from which it recirculates through the tissues and back via the lymph, 'policing' the body for non-self material. Its ability to recognize individual antigens through its specialized surface receptors and to divide into numerous cells of identical specificity and long lifespan makes it the ideal cell for adaptive responses. Two major populations of lymphocytes are recognized: T and B (see also Fig. 15).

B lymphocytes secrete antibody, the humoral element of adaptive immunity.

Antibody is a major fraction of serum proteins, often called immunoglobulin. It is made up of a collection of very similar proteins each able to bind specifically to different antigens, and resulting in a very large repertoire of antigen-binding molecules. Antibodies can bind to and neutralize bacterial toxins and some viruses directly but they also act by **opsonization** and by activating **complement** on the surface of invading pathogens (see below).

T ('thymus-derived') *lymphocytes* are further divided into subpopulations that 'help' B lymphocytes, kill virus-infected cells, activate macrophages and drive inflammation (see Fig. 21).

Interactions between innate and adaptive immunity

Opsonization A phenomenon whereby antibodies bind to the surface of bacteria, viruses or other parasites, and increase their adherence and phagocytosis. Antibody also activates complement on the surface of invading pathogens. Adaptive immunity thus harnesses innate immunity to destroy many microorganisms.

Complement As mentioned above, complement is often activated by antibody bound to microbial surfaces. However, binding of complement to antigen can also greatly increase its ability to activate a strong and lasting B-cell response – an example of 'reverse interaction' between adaptive and innate immune mechanisms.

Presentation of antigens to T and B cells by dendritic cells is necessary for most adaptive responses; presentation by dendritic cells usually requires activation of these cells by contact with microbial components (e.g. bacterial cell walls), another example of 'reverse interaction' between adaptive and innate immune mechanisms.

Help by T cells is required for many branches of both adaptive and innate immunity. T-cell help is required for the secretion of most antibodies by B cells, for activating macrophages to kill intracellular pathogens and for an effective cytotoxic T-cell response.

3 Recognition and receptors: the keys to immunity

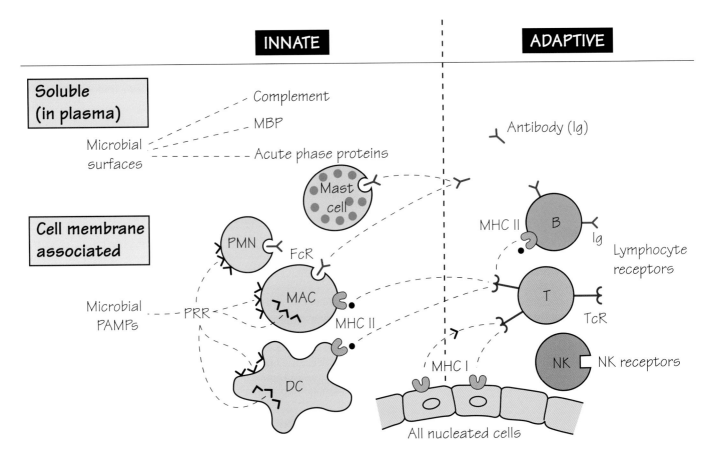

Before any immune mechanism can go into action, there must be a recognition that something exists for it to act against. Normally this means foreign material such as a virus, bacterium or other infectious organism. This recognition is carried out by a series of **recognition molecules or receptors**. Some of these (upper part of figure) circulate freely in blood or body fluids, others are fixed to the membranes of various cells or reside inside the cell cytoplasm (lower part). In every case, some constituent of the foreign material must interact with the recognition molecule like a key fitting into the right lock. This initial act of recognition opens the door that leads eventually to a full **immune response**.

These receptors are quite different in the innate and the adaptive immune system. The innate system (left) possesses a limited number, known as **pattern-recognition receptors** (PRRs), which have been selected during evolution to recognize structures common to groups of disease-causing organisms (pathogen-associated molecular patterns, PAMPs); one example is the lipopolysaccharide (LPS) in some bacterial cell walls (for more details see Fig. 5). These PRRs act as the 'early warning' system of immunity, triggering a rapid inflammatory response (see Fig. 2) which precedes and is essential for a subsequent adaptive response. In contrast, the adaptive system has thousands of millions of different receptors on its B and T lymphocytes (right), each one exquisitely sensitive to one individual molecular structure. The responses triggered by these receptors offer more effective protection against infection, but are usually much slower to develop (see Figs 18–21).

Linking the two systems are the families of major histocompatibility complex (MHC) molecules (centre), specialized for 'serving up' foreign molecules to T lymphocytes. Another set of 'linking' receptors are those by which molecules such as antibody and complement become bound to cells, where they can themselves act as receptors.

 Immunology at a Glance, Tenth Edition. J.H.L. Playfair and B.M. Chain. © 2013 John Wiley & Sons, Ltd. Published 2013 by John Wiley & Sons, Ltd.

Innate immune system
Soluble recognition molecules

Complement A complex set of serum proteins, some of which can be triggered by contact with bacterial surfaces (for details see Fig. 6). Once activated, complement can damage some cells and initiate inflammation. Some cells possess receptors for complement, which can assist the process of phagocytosis (see Fig. 9).

Mannose-binding lectin (MBL) binds the surface of bacteria and fungi, and can activate complement or act directly to assist phagocytosis.

Acute phase proteins Another complex set of serum proteins. Unlike complement, these proteins are mostly present at very low levels in serum, but are rapidly produced in high amounts by the liver following infection, where they contribute to inflammation and immune recognition. Several acute phase proteins also function as **PRR**s.

Cell-associated recognition

PRR Pattern-recognition receptors have now been described for every type of pathogen, and more are being discovered all the time. They can broadly be divided in terms of cellular localization, e.g. cell membrane, endosome/phagosome and cytoplasm. Although they are represented by a bewildering variety of types of molecules, their common functional feature is they regulate the innate immune response to infection. Note that not all PRRs are found on all types of cell, the majority being restricted to macrophages and dendritic cells (MAC, DC in figure). Further details of PRR types are given in Fig. 5.

Some other receptor systems

Receptors feature in a number of other biological processes, many of them outside the scope of this book. Here are a few that are relevant to immunity.

Virus receptors To enter a cell, a virus has to 'dock' with some cell-surface molecule; examples are CD4 for HIV (see Fig. 28) and the acetylcholine receptor for rabies.

Cytokine receptors Communication between immune cells is largely mediated by 'messenger' molecules known as cytokines (see Figs 23 and 24). To respond to a cytokine, a cell needs to possess a receptor for it.

Hormone receptors In the same way as cytokines, hormones (e.g. insulin, steroids) will only act on cells carrying the appropriate receptor.

Adaptive immune system

Antibody Antibody molecules (for details see Figs 13, 14, 19 and 20) can act as both soluble and cell-bound receptors.

1 On the B lymphocyte, antibody molecules synthesized in the cell are exported to the surface membrane where they recognize small components of protein, carbohydrates or other biological macromolecules ('antigens') and are taken into the cell to start the triggering process. Each B lymphocyte is programmed to make antibody of one single recognition type out of a possible hundreds of millions.

2 When the B lymphocyte is triggered, large amounts of its antibody are secreted to act as soluble recognition elements in the blood and tissue fluids; this is referred to as the 'antibody response'. Antibody in serum is often referred to as immunoglobulin (Ig).

3 Some cells possess 'Fc receptors' (FcR in figure) that allow them to take up antibody, insert it in their membrane, and thus become able to recognize a wide range of antigens. This can greatly improve phagocytosis, but can also be responsible for allergies (see Fig. 35).

T-cell receptor (TcR in figure) T lymphocytes carry receptors that have a similar basic structure to antibody on B lymphocytes (for further details see Figs 12 and 18) but with important differences:
1 They are specialized to recognize only small peptides (pieces of proteins) bound to MHC molecules (see below);
2 They are not exported, but act only at the T-cell surface.

MHC molecules These come in two types. MHC class I molecules are expressed on all nucleated cells while class II MHC molecules are normally found only on B lymphocytes, macrophages and dendritic cells. Their role is to 'present' small antigenic peptides to the T-cell receptor. The class of MHC and the type of T cell determine the characteristics of the resulting immune response (see Figs 11 and 18). Their name comes from their important role in stimulating transplant rejection (see Fig. 39).

NK cell receptors Natural killer cells share features of both lymphocytes and innate immune cells. They are specialized for killing virus-infected cells and some tumours, and they possess receptors of two opposing kinds.
1 Activating receptors are analogous to PRRs, recognizing changes associated with stress and virus infection.
2 Inhibitory receptors recognize MHC class I molecules, preventing NK cells killing normal cells. The final result thus depends on the balance between activation and inhibition (for further details see Figs 10, 15 and 42).

LIVERPOOL JOHN MOORES UNIVERSITY
LEARNING SERVICES

4 Cells involved in immunity: the haemopoietic system

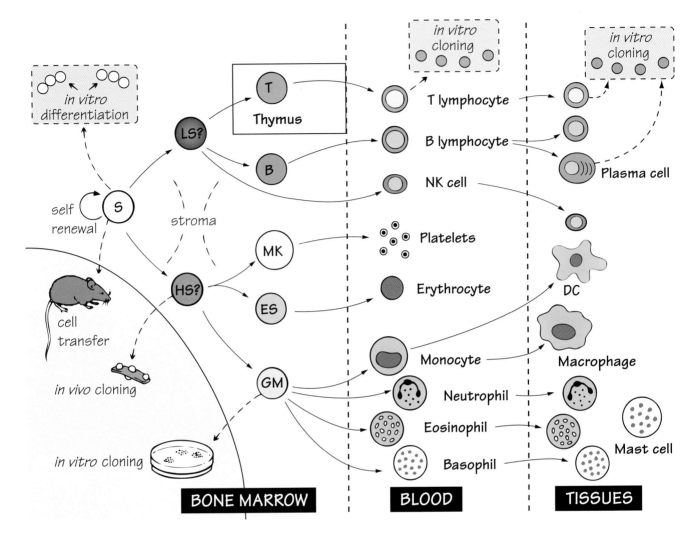

The great majority of cells involved in mammalian immunity are derived from precursors in the **bone marrow** (left half of figure) and circulate in the **blood**, entering and sometimes leaving the **tissues** when required. A very rare stem cell persists in the adult bone marrow (at a frequency of about 1 in 100000 cells), and retains the ability to differentiate into all types of blood cell. Haemopeoisis has been studied either by injecting small numbers of genetically marked marrow cells into recipient mice and observing the progeny they give rise to (*in vivo* cloning) or by culturing the bone marrow precursors in the presence of appropriate growth factors (*in vitro* cloning). Proliferation and differentiation of all these cells is under the control of soluble or membrane-bound **growth factors** produced by the bone marrow stroma and by each other (see Fig. 24). Within the cell these signals switch on specific transcription factors, DNA-binding molecules which act as master switches that determine the subsequent genetic programme, in turn giving rise to development of the different cell types (known as line-

ages). Remarkably, recent studies have shown that it is possible to turn one differentiated cell type into another by experimentally introducing the right transcription factors into the cell. This finding has important therapeutic implications, e.g. in curing genetic immunodeficiencies (see Fig. 33). Most haemopoietic cells stop dividing once they are fully differentiated. However, lymphocytes divide rapidly and expand following exposure to antigen. The increased number of lymphocytes specific for an antigen forms the basis for **immunological memory**.

A note on terminology

Haematologists recognize many stages between stem cells and their fully differentiated progeny (e.g. for red cells: proerythroblast, erythroblast, normoblast, erythrocyte). The suffix '**blast**' usually implies an early, dividing, relatively undifferentiated cell, but is also used to describe lymphocytes that have been stimulated, e.g. by antigen, and are about to divide.

16 *Immunology at a Glance*, Tenth Edition. J.H.L. Playfair and B.M. Chain. © 2013 John Wiley & Sons, Ltd. Published 2013 by John Wiley & Sons, Ltd.

Bone marrow Unlike most other tissues or organs, the haemopoetic system is constantly renewing itself. In the adult, the development of haemopoetic cells occurs predominantly in the bone marrow. In the fetus, before bones develop, haemopoeisis occurs first in the yolk sac and then in the liver.

Stroma Epithelial and endothelial cells that provide support and secrete growth factors for haemopoiesis.

S Stem cell; the totipotent and self-renewing marrow cell. Stem cells are found in low numbers in blood as well as bone marrow and the numbers can be boosted by treatment with appropriate growth factors (e.g. G-CSF), which greatly facilitates the process of bone marrow transplantation (see Fig. 39).

LS Lymphoid stem cell, presumed to be capable of differentiating into T or B lymphocytes. Very recent data suggest that the distinction between lymphoid and myeloid stem cells may in fact be more complex.

HS Haemopoietic stem cell: the precursor of spleen nodules and probably able to differentiate into all but the lymphoid pathways, i.e. granulocyte, erythroid, monocyte, megakaryocyte; often referred to as CFU-GEMM.

ES Erythroid stem cell, giving rise to erythrocytes. Erythropoietin, a glycoprotein hormone formed in the kidney in response to hypoxia, accelerates the differentiation of red cell precursors and thus adjusts the production of red cells to the demand for their oxygen-carrying capacity, a typical example of 'negative feedback'.

GM Granulocyte–monocyte common precursor; the relative proportion of these two cell types is regulated by 'growth-' or 'colony-stimulating' factors (see Fig. 24).

Cloning The potential of individual stem cells to give rise to one or more types of haemopoetic cells has been explored by isolating single cells and allowing them to divide many times, and then observing what cell types can be found among the progeny. This process is known as cloning (a clone being a set of daughter cells all arising from a single parent cell). Evidence suggests that in certain conditions a single stem cell can give rise to all the fully differentiated cells of an adult haemopoetic system.

Neutrophil (polymorph) The most common leucocyte in human blood, a short-lived phagocytic cell whose granules contain numerous bactericidal substances. Neutrophils are the first cells to leave the blood and enter sites of infection or inflammation.

Eosinophil A leucocyte with large refractile granules that contain a number of highly basic or 'cationic' proteins, possibly important in killing larger parasites including worms.

Basophil A leucocyte with large basophilic granules that contain heparin and vasoactive amines, important in the inflammatory response.The above three cell types are often collectively referred to as 'granulocytes'.

MK Megakaryocyte: the parent cell of the blood platelets.

Platelets Small cells responsible for sealing damaged blood vessels ('haemostasis') but also the source of many inflammatory mediators (see Fig. 7).

Monocyte A precursor cell in blood developing into a macrophage when it migrates into the tissues. Additional monocytes are attracted to sites of inflammation, providing a reservoir of macrophages and perhaps also dendritic cells.

Macrophage The principal resident phagocyte of the tissues and serous cavities such as the pleura and peritoneum (see Fig. 8).

DC (dendritic cell) Dendritic cells are found in all tissues of the body (e.g. the Langerhans' cells of the skin) where they take up antigen and then migrate to the T-cell areas of the lymph node or spleen via the lymphatics or the blood. Their major function is to activate T-cell immunity (see Fig. 18), but they may also be involved in tolerance induction (see Fig. 22). A second subset of plasmacytoid DC (a name that derives from their morphological resemblance to plasma cells) are the principal producers of type I interferons, an important group of antiviral proteins. Although experimentally, dendritic cells are often derived from myeloid cells, the developmental lineage of dendritic cells in bone marrow is still the subject of debate.

NK (natural killer) cell A lymphocyte-like cell capable of killing some virus-infected cells and some tumour cells, but with complex sets of receptors that are quite distinct from those on true lymphocytes (for more details see Fig. 10). NK cells and T cells may share a common precursor.

T and B lymphocytes T (thymus-derived) and B (bone marrow-derived or, in birds, bursa-derived) lymphocytes are the major cellular components of adaptive immunity and are described in more detail in Fig. 15. B lymphocytes are the precursor of antibody-forming cells. In fetal life, the liver may play the part of 'bursa'.

Plasma cell A B cell in its high-rate antibody-secreting state. Despite their name, plasma cells are seldom seen in the blood, but are found in spleen, lymph nodes, etc., whenever antibody is being made. Plasma cells do not divide and cannot be maintained for prolonged periods *in vitro*. However, B lymphocytes producing specific antibody can be fused with a tumour cell to produce an immortal hybrid clone or 'hybridoma', which continues to secrete antibody of a predetermined specificity. Such **monoclonal** antibodies have proved of enormous value as specific tools in many branches of biology, and several are now being used routinely for the treatment of autoimmune disease (see Fig. 38) and cancer (see Fig. 42).

Mast cell A large tissue cell derived from the circulating basophil. Mast cells are rapidly triggered by tissue damage to initiate the inflammatory response which causes many forms of allergy (see Fig. 35).

Growth factors The molecules that control the proliferation and differentiation of haemopoietic cells are often also involved in regulating immune responses – the interleukins or cytokines (see Figs 23 and 24). Some of them were first discovered by haematologists and are called 'colony-stimulating factors' (CSF), but the different names have no real significance, and indeed one, IL-3, is often known as 'multi-CSF'. Growth factors are used in clinical practice to boost particular subsets of blood cell, and erythropoietin was one of the first of the new generation of proteins produced by 'recombinant' technology to be used in the clinic, and also by athletes wishing to increase their red cell numbers.

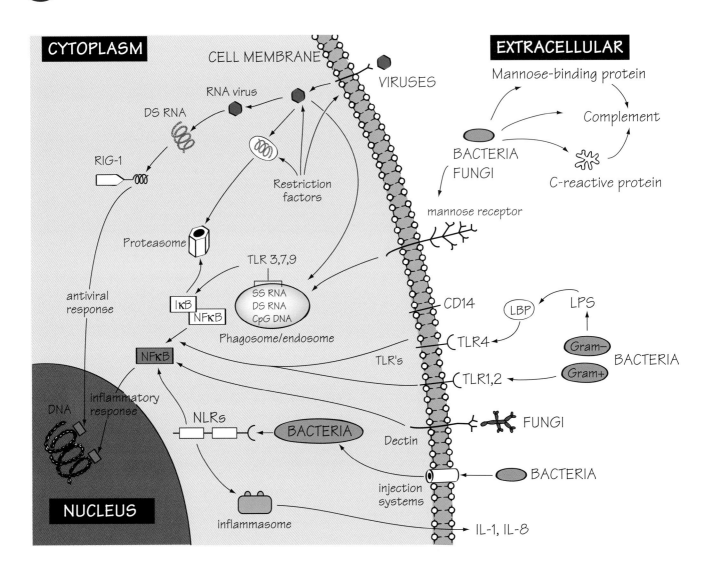

The ability to sense the presence of microorganisms that could cause potentially dangerous infections is a widespread property of cells, tissues and body fluids of all multicellular organisms. This process is called **innate immune recognition.** This recognition process is the first crucial step triggering the complex sequence of events by which the body protects itself against infection. However, it is only since the 1980s that most of the molecules (receptors) responsible for this recognition process have been identified, and new examples of such innate receptors are still being found. The receptors usually recognize components of microorganisms that are not found on cells of the host, e.g. components of bacterial cell wall, bacterial flagella or viral nucleic acids. These target molecules have been named **pathogen-associated**

molecular patterns (PAMPS), and the receptors that recognize them **pattern recognition receptors** (PRRs). Engagement of PRRs by PAMPs results in activation of intracellular signalling pathways, resulting in alteration in gene transcription in the nucleus (left part of figure) and ultimately a whole variety of different cellular responses, broadly termed **inflammation** (illustrated in Fig. 7). Some innate immune receptors are also triggered by damage to cells that arises in the absence of any infection, giving rise to the term damage-associated molecular patterns (DAMPs). The activation of innate immunity is an essential prerequisite for activation for most adaptive immune responses. The major families of PRRs, the structures they recognize and their location within the cell are shown.

Leucine-rich repeats (LRR) A ubiquitous protein structural motif, forming a 'horseshoe'-shaped fold, with an exposed hydrophilic surface and a tightly packed internal hydrophobic core. It is so named because it contains unusually large numbers of the hydrophobic amino acid leucine. LRRs are frequent components of **PRRs**, where they are thought to mediate the interaction between the receptor and the target structure on the microorganism. Families of proteins containing LRRs may also serve primitive antibody-like functions in several types of invertebrates (see Fig. 46).

Toll-like receptors (TLR) Toll-like receptors are so named because of their homology to a gene named *Toll* (from the German word for 'amazing' or 'mad'!) first identified in *Drosphila*. TLRs were the first PRRs to be discovered, and have come to represent the archetype of innate immune recognition receptors. Humans have 10 TLRs, each with an LRR domain involved in recognition of microbial components, and an intracytoplasmic TIR domain involved in signalling into the cell. TLRs associate with a variety of adaptor molecules that help to convert recognition of microbes into a signal, which activates specific gene transcription within the cell.

RIG-1 Many viruses carry their genetic information in the form of RNA, rather than DNA as do all eukaryotes. RIG-1 is an example of a family of molecules that recognize RNA viruses such as influenza, picornaviruses (common cold) and Japanese encephalitis virus, and then switch on the production of **interferons** and other antiviral proteins (see Fig. 23).

Cell surface Innate recognition receptors at the cell surface recognize extracellular microorganisms. The best studied example is TLR4, which together with accessory molecules MD2 and CD14, recognizes lipopolysaccharide (LPS), the principal component of Gram-negative bacterial walls. TLR4 is distributed on many cell types, but is especially important on macrophages (see Figs 7 and 8). Excessive activation of macrophages is thought to be a major factor in **sepsis** and **endotoxic shock,** which leads to oedema and low blood pressure, and can be fatal.

Cytoplasm Many microorganisms can efficiently cross the cellular membrane and colonize the cytoplasm. Viruses are the best known examples of cytoplasmic pathogens. However, many bacteria can also either cross the membrane into the cytoplasm (e.g. *Salmonella*) or can inject toxins and other bacterial components into the cytoplasms. Intracytoplasmic bacterial components are recognized by the **NOD-like receptors**.

NOD-like receptors These are a large family of cytoplasmic proteins that contain **leucine-rich repeats,** which bind to bacterial components. NOD1 and NOD2 recognize fragments of bacterial cell wall proteoglycans, and are found at particularly high amounts in the epithelial cells that line the gut. Mutations in NOD2 have been found to increase the likelihood of developing Crohn's disease, a chronic inflammatory gut disease, perhaps because of a deficient response to bacteria in the gut. Some NOD-like receptors activate the transcription factor **NFκB**. Others activate the **inflammasome.**

The inflammasome This is a multimolecular complex that is assembled in response to triggering of some NOD-like receptors, and leads to the secretion of active forms of the inflammation-promoting cytokines IL-1 and IL-18 (see Fig. 23). Persistent activation of the inflammasome by crystals of uric acid is thought to cause many of the symptoms of gout. In some cases, activation of the inflammasome results in the rapid death of the host cell by a special process known as pyroptosis.

Restriction factors A collection of proteins that inhibit the ability of viruses to replicate. Trim5α binds retroviruses and carries them to the **proteasome**, an intracellular organelle that destroys them. Tetherin, as its name suggests, binds to some viruses as they bud off from the cell surface, limiting the ability of the virus to spread. New restriction factors are continually being discovered.

The endosome/phagosome Many microorganisms are taken up by endocytosis or phagocytosis by macrophages (see Fig. 9). Several TLRs sense microorganisms within these compartments. TLR9 recognizes a type of DNA found predominantly in bacteria and viruses, but rare in eukaryotes (CpG DNA). TLR3 recognizes double-stranded RNA, found in many viruses. TLR7 recognizes single-stranded RNA, which is found in many RNA viruses. Although single-stranded RNA is also a ubiquitous component of eukaryotic cells, it is unstable and cannot survive in the extracellular environment. It therefore seldom enters the endosomal/phagocytic system.

CRP C-reactive protein (MW 130 000), a pentameric globulin (or 'pentraxin') made in the liver which appears in the serum within hours of tissue damage or infection, and whose ancestry goes back to the invertebrates. It binds to phosphorylcholine, which is found on the surface of many bacteria, fixes complement and promotes phagocytosis (see Fig. 6).

Mannose-binding lectin (MBL) A serum protein that binds the sugar mannose, which is often found in large amounts on bacterial or fungal surfaces, but is usually not exposed on mammalian cells. Binding of MBP to microbial surfaces then activates complement (see Fig. 6).

NFκB NFκB is a key transcription factor regulating the inflammatory response. Normally, it is kept inactive in the **cytoplasm** by binding to the inhibitor IκB. However, activation of many **PRRs** (see figure) results in destruction of IκB by the **proteasome**, and NFκB then moves into the nucleus where it switches on many components of the antibacterial, antiviral and inflammatory response.

Proteasome A cytoplasmic organelle whose major function is to break down proteins and recycle their constituent amino acids within the cell. It also has a key role in producing the peptides recognized by the T lymphocyte (see Fig. 18).

Dectin-1 and the mannose receptor These are just two members of an enormous family of sugar-binding proteins known as C-type lectins. They have an important role in binding to fungal and bacterial cell walls, activating phagocytosis and inflammation (see Figs 8 and 9).

6 Complement

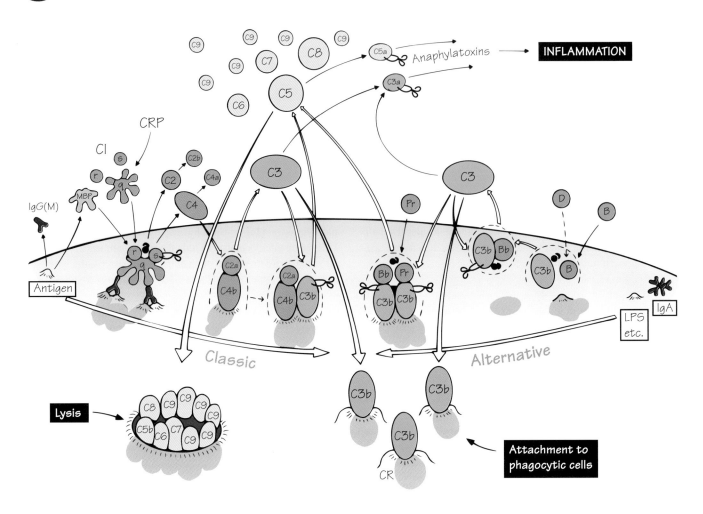

Fifteen or more serum components constitute the **complement** system, the sequential activation and assembly into functional units of which leads to three main effects: release of peptides active in **inflammation** (top right); deposition of C3b, a powerful attachment promoter (or 'opsonin') for **phagocytosis**, on cell membranes (bottom right); and membrane damage resulting in **lysis** (bottom left). Together these make it an important part of the defences against microorganisms. Deficiencies of some components can predispose to severe infections, particularly bacterial (see Fig. 33).

The upper half of the figure represents the serum, or 'fluid' phase, the lower half the cell surface, where activation (indicated by dotted haloes) and assembly largely occur. Activation of complement can be started either via adaptive or innate immune recognition. The former pathway is called '**classic**' (because first described), and is initiated by the binding of specific antibody of the IgG or IgM class (see Fig. 14) to surface antigens (centre left); the innate, and probably earlier evolutionary pathways include the '**alternative**' pathway, in which complement components are activated by direct interaction with polysaccharides on some microbial cell surfaces, or by a variety of

pattern recognition receptors (PRRs; see Fig. 5) including '**mannose-binding lectin** (MBL) and C-reactive protein (CRP; centre left). Some of the steps are dependent on the divalent ions Ca^{2+} (shaded circles) or Mg^{2+} (black circles). A key feature of complement is that it functions via a biochemical **cascade**: a single activation event (whether by antibody or via innate pathways) leads to the production of many downstream events, such as deposition of C3b.

Activation is usually limited to the immediate vicinity by the very short life of the active products, and in some cases there are special inactivators (represented here by scissors). Nevertheless, excessive complement activation can cause unpleasant side-effects (see Fig. 36).

Note that, in the absence of antibody, many of the molecules that activate the complement system are carbohydrate or lipid in nature (e.g. lipopolysaccharides, mannose), suggesting that the system evolved mainly to recognize bacterial surfaces via their non-protein features. With the appearance of antibody in the vertebrates (see Fig. 46), it became possible for virtually any foreign molecule to activate the system.

Classic pathway

For many years this was the only way in which complement was known to be activated. The essential feature is the requirement for a specific antigen–antibody interaction, leading via components C1, C2 and C4 to the formation of a 'convertase' which splits C3.

Ig IgM and some subclasses of IgG (in the human, IgG1–IgG3), when bound to antigen are recognized by C1q to initiate the classic pathway.

C1 A Ca^{2+}-dependent union of three components: C1q (MW 400 000), a curious protein with six valencies for Ig linked by collagen-like fibrils, which activates in turn C1r (MW 170 000) and C1s (MW 80 000), a serine proteinase that goes on to attack C2 and C4.

C2 (MW 120 000), split by C1s into small (C2b) and large (C2a) fragments.

C4 (MW 240 000), likewise split into C4a (small) and C4b (large). C4b then binds to C2, and also, via a very unusual type of reactive thioester bond, to any local macromolecule, such as the antigen–antibody complex itself, or to the membrane in the case of a cell-bound antigen. This tethers the C4bC2 complex forming a 'C3 convertase'. Note that some complementologists prefer to reverse the names of C2a and b, so that for both C2 and C4 the 'a' peptide is the smaller one.

C3 (MW 180 000), the central component of all complement reactions, split by its convertase into a small (C3a) and a large (C3b) fragment. Some of the C3b is deposited on the membrane, where it serves as an attachment site for phagocytic polymorphs and macrophages, which have receptors for it; some remains associated with C2a and C4b, forming a 'C5 convertase'. Two 'C3b inactivator' enzymes rapidly inactivate C3b, releasing the fragment C3c and leaving membrane-bound C3d.

C5 (MW 180 000), split by its convertase into C5a, a small peptide that, together with C3a (anaphylatoxins), acts on mast cells, polymorphs and smooth muscle to promote the inflammatory response, and C5b, which initiates the assembly of C6, 7, 8 and 9 into the membrane-damaging or 'lytic' unit.

CR Complement receptor. Three types of molecule that bind different products of C3 breakdown are found on cell surfaces: CR1 is found on red cells, and is important for the removal of antibody–antigen complexes from blood; CR1 and CR3 on phagocytic cells, where they act as opsonins (see Fig. 9); and CR2 on B lymphocytes where it has a role in enhancing antibody production but is also, unfortunately, the receptor via which the Epstein–Barr virus (glandular fever) gains entry (see Fig. 27).

Alternative pathway

The principal features distinguishing this from the classic pathway are the lack of dependence on calcium ions and the lack of need for C1, C2 or C4, and therefore for specific antigen–antibody interaction. Instead, several different molecules can initiate C3 conversion, notably lipopolysaccharides (LPS) and other bacterial products, but also including aggregates of some types of antibody such as IgA (see Fig. 20). Essentially, the alternative pathway consists of a continuously 'ticking over' cycle, held in check by control molecules, the effects of which are counteracted by the various initiators.

B Factor B (MW 100 000), which complexes with C3b, whether produced via the classic pathway or the alternative pathway itself. It has both structural and functional similarities to C2, and both are coded for by genes within the very important major histocompatibility complex (see Fig. 11). In birds, which lack C2 and C4, C1 activates factor B.

D Factor D (MW 25 000), an enzyme that acts on the C3b–B complex to produce the active convertase, referred to in the language of complementologists as C3bBb.

Pr Properdin (MW 220 000), the first isolated component of the alternative pathway, once thought to be the actual initiator but now known merely to stabilize the C3b–B complex so that it can act on further C3. Thus, more C3b is produced which, with factors B and D, leads in turn to further C3 conversion, a 'positive feedback' loop with great amplifying potential (but restrained by the C3b inactivators factor H and factor I).

MBL and other pathways

MBL Mannose-binding lectin (also variously referred to as mannose-binding protein or mannan-binding protein), a C1q-like molecule that recognizes microbial components such as yeast mannan and activates C1r and C1s, and hence the rest of the classic pathway. MBL deficiency predisposes children to an increased incidence of some bacterial infections.

CRP C-reactive protein, produced in large amounts during 'acute-phase' responses (see Fig. 7), binds to bacterial phosphorylcholine and activates C1q.

Lytic pathway

Lysis of cells is probably the least vital of the complement reactions, but one of the easiest to study. It is initiated by the splitting of C5 by one of its two convertases: C3b–C2a–C4b (classic pathway) or C3b–Bb–Pr (alternative pathway). Thereafter the results are the same, however caused.

C6 (MW 150 000), **C7** (MW 140 000) and **C8** (MW 150 000) unite with C5b, one molecule of each, and with 10 or more molecules of **C9** (MW 80 000). This 'membrane attack complex' is shaped somewhat like a cylindrical tube and when inserted into the membrane of bacteria, red cells, etc. causes leakage of the contents and death by lysis. Needless to say, some bacteria have evolved various strategies for avoiding this (see Fig. 29).

Complement inhibitors

In order to prevent over-activation of the complement cascade, there are numerous inhibitory mechanisms regulating complement. Some of these, like C1q inhibitor, block the activity of complement proteinases. Others cleave active complement components into inactive fragments (factor I). Yet others destabilize the molecular complexes that build up during complement activation. Genetic manipulation has been used to make pigs carrying a transgene coding for the human version of one such important regulatory protein, DAF (decay accelerating factor); results suggest that tissues from such pigs are less rapidly rejected when transplanted into primates, increasing the chances of carrying out successful xenotransplantation (see Fig. 39).

7 Acute inflammation

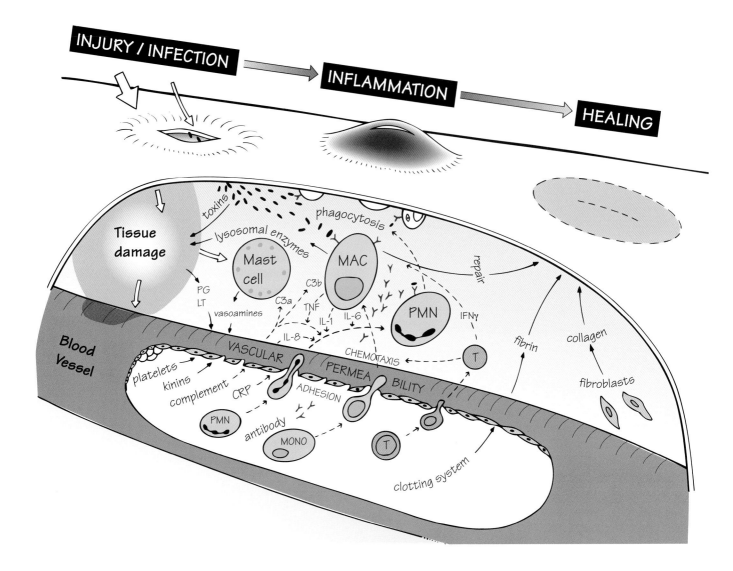

Whether **inflammation** should be considered part of immunology is a problem for the teaching profession, not for the body, which combats infection by all the means at its disposal, including mechanisms also involved in the response to, and repair of, other types of damage.

In this simplified scheme, which should be read from left to right, are shown the effects of **injury** to tissues (top left) and to blood vessels (bottom left). The small black rods represent bacterial **infection**, a very common cause of inflammation and of course a frequent accompaniment of injury. Note the central role of **permeability of the vascular endothelium** in allowing access of blood cells and serum components (lower half) to the tissues (upper half), which also accounts for the main symptoms of inflammation – redness, warmth, swelling and pain.

It can be seen that the 'adaptive' (or 'immunological') functions of antibody and lymphocytes largely operate to amplify or focus pre-existing 'innate' mechanisms; quantitatively, however, they are so important that they frequently make the difference between life and death. Further details of the role of antibody and lymphocytes in inflammation can be found in Figs 34–39.

Note the central importance of the tissue **mast cells** and **macrophages**, and the blood-derived **PMNs**. Inflammation is usually localized to the area of injury or infection. Occasionally, e.g. in sepsis, uncontrolled inflammation becomes systemic, and causes severe illness, organ failure and ultimately death. Sepsis remains a serious risk after major surgery. If for any reason inflammation does not die down within a matter of days, it may become chronic, and here the macrophage and the T lymphocyte have dominant roles (see Fig. 37).

Mast cell A large tissue cell with basophilic granules containing vasoactive amines and heparin. It degranulates readily in response to injury by trauma, heat, ultraviolet light, etc. and also in some allergic conditions (see Fig. 35).

PG, LT Prostaglandins and leukotrienes: a family of unsaturated fatty acids (MW 300–400) derived by metabolism of arachidonic acid, a component of most cell membranes. Individual PGs and LTs have different but overlapping effects; together they are responsible for the induction of pain, fever, vascular permeability and chemotaxis of PMNs, and some of them also inhibit lymphocyte functions. Aspirin, paracetamol and other non-steroidal anti-inflammatory drugs act principally by blocking PG production.

Vasoamines Vasoactive amines, e.g. histamine and 5-hydroxytryptamine, produced by mast cells, basophils and platelets, and causing increased capillary permeability.

Kinin system A series of serum peptides sequentially activated to cause vasodilatation and increased permeability.

Complement A cascading sequence of serum proteins, activated either directly ('alternate pathway') or via antigen–antibody interaction (for details see Fig. 6).

C3a and C5a These stimulate release by mast cells of their vasoactive amines, and are known as anaphylatoxins.

Opsonization C3b attached to a particle promotes sticking to phagocytic cells because of their 'C3 receptors'. Antibody, if present, augments this by binding to 'Fc receptors'.

CRP C-reactive protein (MW 130000), a pentameric globulin (or 'pentraxin') made in the liver which appears in the serum within hours of tissue damage or infection, and whose ancestry goes back to the invertebrates. It binds to phosphorylcholine, which is found on the surface of many bacteria, fixes complement and promotes phagocytosis; thus it may have an antibody-like role in some bacterial infections. Proteins whose serum concentration increases during inflammation are called '**acute-phase proteins**'; they include CRP and many complement components, as well as other microbe-binding molecules and enzyme inhibitors. This **acute-phase response** can be viewed as a rapid, not very specific, attempt to deal with more or less any type of infection or damage.

PMN Polymorphonuclear leucocyte; the major mobile phagocytic cell, whose prompt arrival in the tissues plays a vital part in removing invading bacteria.

Mono Monocyte: the precursor of tissue macrophages (MAC in the figure) that is responsible for removing damaged tissue as well as microorganisms. The tissue macrophages are also an important source of the inflammatory cytokines tumour necrosis factor α (TNF-α), IL-1 and IL-6 (see below).

Lysosomal enzymes Bactericidal enzymes released from the lysosomes of PMNs, monocytes and macrophages, e.g. lysozyme, myeloperoxidase and others, also capable of damaging normal tissues.

Inflammatory cytokines The inflammatory response is orchestrated by several cytokines, which are produced by a variety of cell types. The most important are TNF-α, IL-6 and IL-1. All these cytokines have many functions (they are 'pleiotropic'), including initiating many of the changes in the vascular endothelium that promote leucocyte entry into the inflammatory site. They also induce the acute phase response and, later, the process of tissue repair. IL-1 is one of the few cytokines that acts systemically, rather than locally; e.g. through its action on the hypothalamus, it is the main molecule responsible for inducing fever. See Figs 23 and 24 for further details of cytokines.

Chemotaxis C5a, C3a, leukotrienes and 'chemokines' stimulate PMNs and monocytes to move into the tissues. Movement towards the site of inflammation is called chemotaxis, and is due to the cells' ability to detect a concentration gradient of chemotactic factors; random increases of movement are called chemokinesis.

Chemokines These are a very large family of small polypeptides, which have a key role in chemotaxis and the regulation of leucocyte trafficking. There are two main classes of chemokines, based on the distribution of conserved disulphide bonds. They bind to an equally large family of chemokine receptors, and the biology of the system is further complicated by the fact that many of the chemokines have multiple functions, and can bind to many different receptors. Although some have been called interleukins (e.g. IL-8), the majority have retained separate names. They shot to prominence when it was discovered that some of the chemokine receptors (e.g. CCR5 receptor) served as essential coreceptors (together with CD4) for HIV to gain entry into cells (see Fig. 28).

Adhesion and cell traffic Changes in the expression of endothelial surface molecules, induced mainly by cytokines, cause PMNs, monocytes and lymphocytes to slow down and subsequently adhere to the vessel wall. These 'adhesion molecules' and the molecules they bind to fall into well-defined groups (selectins, integrins, the Ig superfamily; see Fig. 10). These changes, together with the selective local release of **chemokines**, regulate the changes in cell traffic that underlie all inflammatory responses.

T lymphocyte T lymphocyte, undergoing proliferation and activation when stimulated by antigen, as is the case in most infections. By releasing cytokines such as interferon-γ (IFN-γ) (see Figs 23, 24), T cells can greatly increase the activity of macrophages.

Clotting system Intimately bound up with complement and kinins because of several shared activation steps. Blood clotting is a vital part of the healing process.

Fibrin The end product of blood clotting and, in the tissues, the matrix into which fibroblasts migrate to initiate healing.

Fibroblast An important tissue cell that migrates into the fibrin clot and secretes **collagen**, an enormously strong polymerizing molecule giving the healing wound its strength and elasticity. Subsequently new blood capillaries sprout into the area, leading eventually to restoration of the normal architecture.

8 Phagocytic cells and the reticuloendothelial system

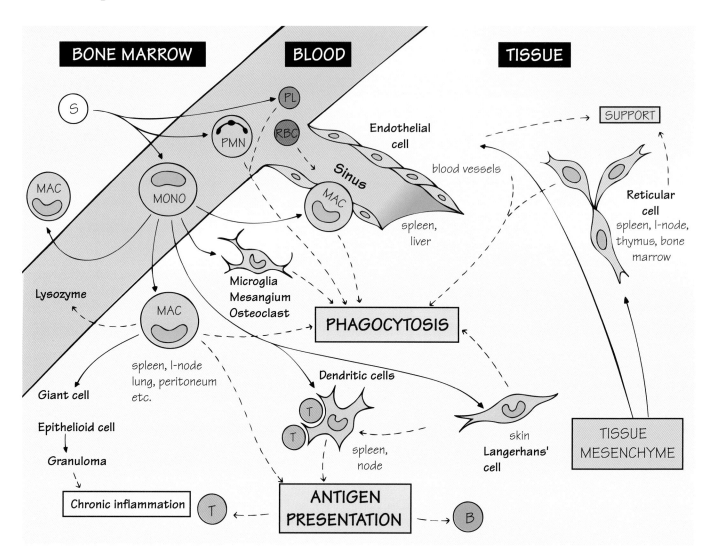

Particulate matter that finds its way into the blood or tissues is rapidly removed by cells, and the property of taking up dyes, colloids, etc. was used by anatomists to define a body-wide system of **phagocytic** cells known as the '**reticuloendothelial system**' (RES), consisting of the vascular endothelium and reticular tissue cells (top right), and – supposedly descended from these – various types of macrophages with routine functions that included clearing up the body's own debris and killing and digesting bacteria.

However, more modern work has shown a fundamental distinction between those phagocytic cells derived from the bone marrow (blue in figure) and endothelial and reticular cells formed locally from the tissues themselves (yellow). Ironically, neither reticular nor endothelial cells are outstandingly phagocytic. Their function is partly structural, in maintaining the integrity of the lymphoid tissue and blood vessels, respectively. However, there is increasing awareness that both

cell types have an equally important role as 'signposts', regulating the migration of haemopoietic cells from blood into the tissues and through the various subcompartments of lymphoid tissue.

In contrast, the major phagocytic tissue cell is the macrophage, and it is therefore more usual today to speak of the '**mononuclear phagocytic system**' (MPS). The cells of the MPS are now recognized as fundamental to both the 'recognition' and the 'mopping up' phase of the adaptive immune response (see Fig. 1). Macrophages and dendritic cells act as tissue sentinels, responding to infection and tissue damage via 'innate' receptors (see Fig. 5) and signalling the alarm to adaptive immunity via both antigen presentation (see Fig. 18) and the release of powerful cytokines. Once an adaptive immune response is established, one of the main roles of antibody is to promote and amplify phagocytosis, while T lymphocytes serve to activate macrophage microbicidal activity (see Figs 21 and 37).

Endothelial cell The inner lining of blood vessels, able to take up dyes, etc. but not truly phagocytic. Endothelial cells direct the passage of leucocytes from blood into tissues, and can both produce and respond to cytokines rather as macrophages do. They can also present antigen directly to T cells under some circumstances.

Reticular cell The main supporting or 'stromal' cell of lymphoid organs, usually associated with the collagen-like reticulin fibres, and not easily distinguished from fibroblasts or from other branching or 'dendritic' cells (see below) – whence a great deal of confusion.

Mesangium Mesangial cells are specialized macrophages found in the kidney, where they phagocytose material deposited in it, particularly complexes of antigen and antibody (see Fig. 36).

Osteoclast A large multinucleate macrophage responsible for resorbing and so shaping bone and cartilage. It is regulated by cytokines such as TNF-α and IL-1, and is thought to have a role in degenerative diseases of joints such as rheumatoid arthritis.

Dendritic cells The weakly phagocytic **Langerhans' cell** of the epidermis, and somewhat similar cells in other tissues migrate through the lymphatic vessels (where they are known as 'veiled' cells) or blood to lymph nodes and spleen, where they are the main agents of T-cell stimulation; T cells recognize foreign antigens in association with cell-surface antigens coded for by the MHC, a genetic region intimately involved in immune responses of all kinds (see Figs 11, 12 and 18). The precursor of the dendritic cell comes from the bone marrow (see Fig. 4) but its precise lineage remains controversial. There are separate follicular dendritic cells for presenting antigen to B cells that specialize in trapping antigen–antibody complexes. They are found in the B-cell areas of lymphoid tissue (see Figs 17 and 19), but are one of the very few cells of the immune system that are not derived from bone marrow, being of fibroblast origin.

Kupffer cells Specialized macrophages found in the liver where they remove dying or damaged red blood cells and other material from the circulation. They make up a major fraction of the phagocytic cells in the body.

T and B Lymphocytes are often found in close contact with dendritic cells; this is presumably where antigen presentation and T–B cell cooperation take place (see Figs 18 and 19).

S The totipotent bone marrow stem cell, giving rise to all the cells found in blood (see Fig. 4).

PL Blood platelets, although primarily involved in clotting, are able to phagocytose antigen–antibody complexes, and can also secrete some cytokines, such as transforming growth factor β (TGF-β).

RBC Antigen–antibody complexes that have bound complement can become attached to red blood cells via the CR1 receptor (see Fig. 6) which then transport the complexes to the liver for removal by macrophages. This is sometimes referred to as 'immune adherence'.

PMN Polymorphonuclear leucocyte, the major phagocytic cell of the blood; however, not conventionally considered as part of the MPS.

MONO Monocyte, formed in the bone marrow and travelling via the blood to the tissues, where it matures into a macrophage. Some monocytes patrol the surface of blood vessels, presumably to repair sites of damage or infection.

MAC Macrophage, the resident and long-lived tissue phagocyte (see Fig. 9). Macrophages may be either free in the tissues, or 'fixed' in the walls of blood sinuses, where they monitor the blood for particles, effete red cells, etc. Macrophages in the lung alveoli (alveolar macrophages) are responsible for keeping these vital air sacs free of particles and microbes. Macrophages (and polymorphs) have the valuable ability to recognize not only foreign matter, but also antibody and/or complement bound to it, which greatly enhances phagocytosis. Despite their important role in host defence, the over-activation of macrophages and particularly their ability to produce high levels of reactive oxygen intermediates and the inflammatory cytokine TNF-α, is increasingly recognized as playing an important part in a very wide variety of chronic inflammatory conditions, including such common diseases as rheumatoid arthritis, psoriasis, Alzheimer's disease and atherosclerosis.

Antibody-mediated cellular cytotoxicity (ADCC) Monocytes, macrophages and granulocytes can all kill target cells by a process similar to that of CD8 cytotoxic T cells (see Fig. 21) but it is mediated by an antibody-mediated interaction (ADCC).

Sinus Tortuous channels in liver, spleen, etc. through which blood passes to reach the veins, allowing the lining macrophages to remove damaged or antibody-coated cells and other particles. This process is so effective that a large injection of, for example, carbon particles can be removed from the blood within minutes, leaving the liver and spleen visibly black.

Microglia The phagocytic cells of the brain, implicated in tissue injury leading to Alzheimer's disease and multiple sclerosis. Unlike other tissue macrophages, microglia may be derived from a special precursor cell that enters the brain before birth and divides within the brain.

Lysozyme An important antibacterial enzyme secreted into the blood by macrophages. Macrophages also produce other 'innate' humoral factors such as interferon and many complement components, cytotoxic factors, etc.

Giant cell; epithelioid cell Macrophage-derived cells typically found at sites of chronic inflammation; by coalescing into a solid mass, or **granuloma**, they localize and wall off irritant or indigestible materials (see Fig. 37). However, granulomas also have a major role in disease (e.g. in tuberculosis) by obstructing airways and causing internal bleeding.

9 Phagocytosis

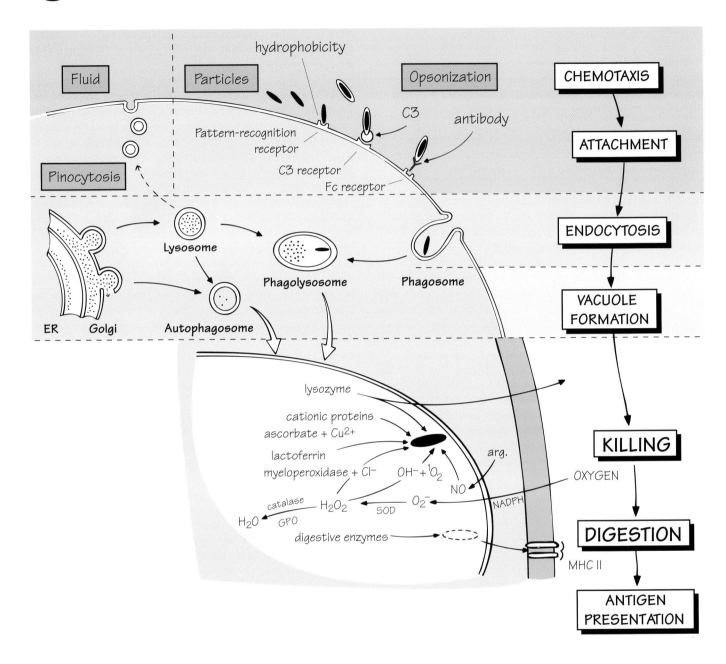

Numerous cells are able to ingest foreign materials, but the ability to increase this activity in response to opsonization by antibody and/or complement, so as to acquire antigen specificity, is restricted to cells of the myeloid series, principally **polymorphs**, **monocytes** and **macrophages**; these are sometimes termed 'professional' phagocytes.

Apart from some variations in their content of lysosomal enzymes, all these cells use essentially similar mechanisms to phagocytose foreign objects, consisting of a sequence of **attachment** (top), endocytosis or **ingestion** (centre) and **digestion** (bottom). In the figure this process is shown for a typical bacterium (small black rods). In general, bacteria with **capsules** (shown as a white outline) are not phagocytosed unless opsonized, whereas many non-capsulated ones do not require this. There are certain differences between phagocytic cells; e.g. polymorphs are very short-lived (hours or days) and often die in the process of phagocytosis, while macrophages, which lack some of the more destructive enzymes, usually survive to phagocytose again. Also, macrophages can actively secrete some of their enzymes, e.g. lysozyme. There are surprisingly large species differences in the proportions of the various lysosomal enzymes.

Several of the steps in phagocytosis shown in the figure may be specifically defective for genetic reasons (see Fig. 33), as well as being actively inhibited by particular microorganisms (see Figs 27–32). In either case the result is a failure to eliminate microorganisms or foreign material properly, leading to chronic infection and/or chronic inflammation.

Chemotaxis The process by which cells are attracted towards bacteria, etc., often by following a gradient of molecules released by the microbe (see Fig. 7).

Pinocytosis 'Cell drinking'; the ingestion of soluble materials, including water, conventionally applied also to particles under 1 μm in diameter.

Hydrophobicity Hydrophobic groups tend to attach to the hydrophobic surface of cells; this may explain the 'recognition' of damaged cells, denatured proteins, etc. (see Fig. 29).

Pattern-recognition receptors Phagocytic cells have surface and phagosomal receptors that recognize complementary molecular structures on the surface of common pathogens (for details see Fig. 5). Binding between pathogens and these receptors activates intracellular killing and digestion, as well as the release of many inflammatory chemokines and cytokines (see Figs 23 and 24).

C3 receptor Phagocytic cells (and some lymphocytes) can bind C3b, produced from C3 by activation by bacteria, etc., either directly or via antibody (for details of the receptors see Fig. 6).

Fc receptor Phagocytic cells (and some lymphocytes, platelets, etc.) can bind the Fc portion of antibody, especially of the IgG class. Binding of several IgG molecules to Fc receptors on macrophages or polymorphs triggers receptor activation, and activates phagocytosis and microbial killing.

Opsonization This refers to the promotion or enhancement of attachment via the C3 or Fc receptor. Discovered by Almroth Wright and made famous by G.B. Shaw in *The Doctor's Dilemma*, opsonization is probably the single most important process by which antibody helps to overcome infections, particularly bacterial.

Phagosome A vacuole formed by the internalization of surface membrane along with an attached particle. The phagosome often fuses with the lysosome, thus exposing the internalized microorganism to the destructive power of the lysosomal enzymes or cathepsins. However, some pathogens (e.g. some species of *Salmonella*) have evolved ways to avoid phagolysosome fusion, and thus survive within the phagocyte unharmed.

Microtubules Short rigid structures composed of the protein tubulin which arrange themselves into channels for vacuoles, etc. to travel within the cell.

Microfilaments Contractile protein (actin) filaments responsible for membrane activities such as pinocytosis and phagosome formation. There are also intermediate filaments composed of the protein vimentin.

ER Endoplasmic reticulum: a membranous system of sacs and tubules with which ribosomes are associated in the synthesis of many proteins for secretion.

Golgi The region where products of the ER are packaged into vesicles (see also Fig. 19).

Lysosome A membrane-bound package of hydrolytic enzymes usually active at acid pH (e.g. acid phosphatase, DNAase). Lysosomes are found in almost all cells, and are vehicles for secretion as well as digestion. They are prominent in macrophages and polymorphs, which also have separate vesicles containing lysozyme and other enzymes; together with lysosomes these constitute the **granules** whose staining patterns characterize the various types of polymorph (neutrophil, basophil, eosinophil). Genetic defects in specific lysosomal enzymes can result in serious or even fatal lysosomal storage diseases, such as Tay–Sachs, or Gaucher's disease.

Phagolysosome A vacuole formed by the fusion of a phagosome and lysosome(s), in which microorganisms are killed and digested. The pH is tightly controlled, and varies between different phagocytes, presumably so as to maximize the activity of different types of lysosomal enzymes.

Autophagy Literally, 'eating oneself', this refers to a process whereby cells can sequester cytoplasm or organelles into newly formed membrane vesicles, to form **autophagosomes**, which then fuse with lysosomes and degrade the contents. It is stimulated by cell stress or starvation, but also by activation of many innate immune receptors (see Fig. 5). Autophagy is an important mechanisms for cells to turn over old or damaged proteins and organelles, and may function as an additional source of energy when cells are stressed or damaged. Autophagy is also important in resistance to some microorganisms, including tuberculosis, although the mechanisms remain unclear (see Fig. 18).

Lactoferrin A protein that inhibits bacteria by depriving them of iron, which it binds with an extremely high affinity.

Cationic proteins Examples are 'phagocytin', 'leukin'; microbicidal agents found in some polymorph granules. Eosinophils are particularly rich in cationic proteins, which can be secreted when the cell 'degranulates', making them highly cytotoxic cells.

Ascorbate Ascorbate interacts with copper ions and hydrogen peroxide, and can be bactericidal.

Oxygen and the oxygen burst Intracellular killing of many bacteria requires the uptake of oxygen by the phagocytic cell, i.e. it is 'aerobic'. Through a series of enzyme reactions including NADPH oxidase and superoxide dismutase (SOD), this oxygen is progressively reduced to superoxide (O_2^-), hydrogen peroxide (H_2O_2), hydroxyl ions (OH^-) and singlet oxygen ($^1O_2$). These reactive oxygen species (ROS) are rapidly removed by cellular enzymes such as **catalase** and glutathione peroxidase. ROS are highly toxic to many microorganisms but excessive ROS production may contribute to damage to host tissues, e.g. blood vessels in arteriosclerosis.

NO Nitric oxide produced from arginine is another reactive oxygen-containing compound that is highly toxic to microorganisms when produced in large amounts by activated mouse macrophages; its importance in humans remains less well established. In contrast, much lower levels of nitric oxide are produced constitutively by endothelial cells, and have a key role in the regulation of blood vessel tone.

Myeloperoxidase An important enzyme of PMNs that converts hydrogen peroxide and halide (e.g. chloride) ions into the microbicide hypochlorous acid (bleach). Reaction of antigens with hypochlorous acid may also enhance their recognition by T lymphocytes.

Lysozyme (muramidase) This lyses many saprophytes (e.g. *Micrococcus lysodeicticus*) and some pathogenic bacteria damaged by antibody and/or complement. It is a major secretory product of macrophages, present in the blood at levels of micrograms per millilitre.

Digestive enzymes The enzymes by which lysosomes are usually identified, such as acid phosphatase, lipase, elastase, β-glucuronidase and the cathepsins, some of which are thought to be important in antigen processing via the **MHC** class II pathway (see Fig. 18).

10 Evolution of recognition molecules: the immunoglobulin superfamily

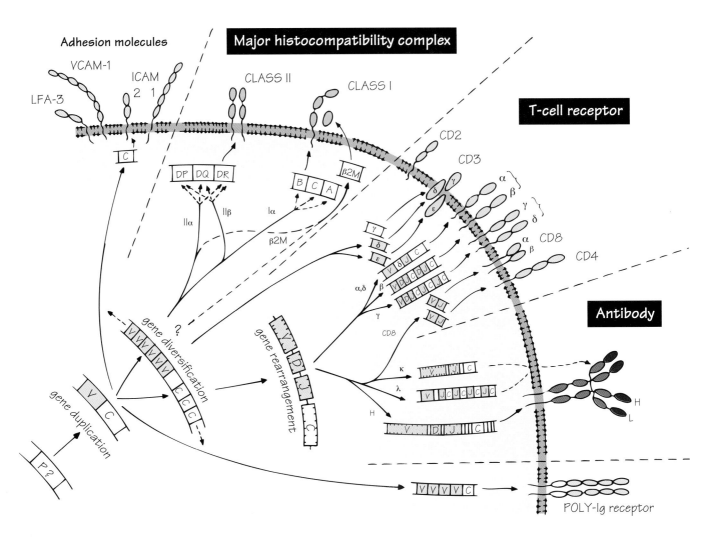

At this point it may be worth re-emphasizing the difference between 'innate' and 'adaptive' immunity, which lies essentially in the degree of **discrimination** of the respective recognition systems.

Innate immune recognition, e.g. by phagocytic cells, NK cells or the alternative complement pathway, uses a limited number of different receptors (more are being discovered all the time, but there are probably only a few dozen in total), which have evolved to recognize directly the most important classes of pathogen (see Figs 3 and 5).

Recognition by **lymphocytes**, the fundamental cells of adaptive immunity, is quite another matter. An enormous range of foreign substances can be individually distinguished and the appropriate response set in motion. This is only possible because of the evolution of three sets of **cell-surface receptors**, each showing extensive heterogeneity, namely the **antibody** molecule, the **T-cell receptor** and the molecules of the **major histocompatibility complex** (MHC). Thanks to molecular biology, the fascinating discovery was made that all these receptors share enough sequences, at both the gene (DNA) and protein

(amino acid) level, to make it clear that they have evolved from a single precursor, presumably a primitive recognition molecule of some kind (see Figs 3 and 46). The three-dimensional structure of all these receptors which was obtained more recently using X-ray crystallography has confirmed this close relationship.

Because antibody was the first of these genetic systems to be identified, they are often collectively referred to as the **immunoglobulin gene superfamily**, which contains other related molecules too, some with immunological functions, some without. What they all share is a structure based on a number of folded sequences about 110 amino acids long and featuring β-pleated sheets, called **domains** (shown in the figure as oval loops protruding from the cell membrane).

Much work is still needed to fill in the evolutionary gaps, and the figure can only give an impression of what the relationships between this remarkable family of molecules may have been. Their present-day structure and function are considered in more detail in the following four figures.

P? The precursor gene from which the immunoglobulin superfamily is presumed to have evolved. It is believed that the key to the evolutionary success of the characteristic immunoglobulin **domain** is its extreme resistance to chemical or physical destruction. The gene has not been identified in any existing species, but may well have coded for a molecule that mediated cell–cell recognition. Alternative mechanisms for generating very diverse families of recognition molecules have been discovered very recently in several invertebrates and primitive vertebrates, some of which seem to be based on the leucine-rich repeat (LRR) protein domain instead of the immunoglobulin domain (see Fig. 5).

V, C A vital early step seems to have been the duplication of this gene into two, one of which became the parent of all present-day **variable** (V) genes and the other of **constant** (C) genes. In the figure, the genes and polypeptides with sufficient homology to be considered part of the V gene family are shown in blue. Subsequent further duplications, with diversification among different V and C genes, led ultimately to the large variety of present-day domains.

Major histocompatibility complex The genes shown are those found in humans, also known as HLA (human leucocyte antigen) genes. Interactions between MHC molecules and T-cell receptors are vital to all adaptive immune responses. Further details are shown in Fig. 11.

β2M β$_2$-Microglobulin, which combines with class I chains to complete the four-domain molecule.

Gene rearrangement A process found only in T and B cells, through which an enormous degree of receptor diversity is generated by bringing together one V gene and one J gene (and one D gene in the case of IgH chains), each from a set containing from 2 to over 100. The joins between the segments are imprecise, leading to millions of possible receptors (see Figs 12 and 13). This unique process of chromosomal gene rearrangement is brought about by enzymes called recombinases.

T-cell receptor (TCR) A complex of T-cell surface molecules, including TCR α plus β, or γ plus δ chains, CD3 and CD4 or CD8, depending on the type of T cell. Together these form a unit that enables the T cell to recognize a specific antigen plus a particular MHC molecule, to become activated and to carry out its function (help, cytotoxicity, etc.; for more details see Fig. 12).

Antibody The antibody or immunoglobulin molecule plays the part of cell-surface receptor on B lymphocytes as well as being secreted in vast amounts by activated B cells to give rise to serum antibody, a vital part of defence against infectious organisms. The domains are fairly similar to those of the TCR α and β chains, but assembled in a different way, with two four-domain heavy (H) chains bonded to two two-domain light (L) chains (see Figs 13 and 14).

Note that the process of diversification in the genes for the various chains has not always proceeded in the same way. For example, mammalian heavy and light (κ) chains have all their J genes together, between V and C, while light (λ) chains have repeated J–C segments and sharks have the whole V–D–J–C segment duplicated, a considerably less efficient arrangement for generating the maximum diversity.

Costimulatory molecules T-cell proliferation and cytokine release (see Fig. 21) is governed both by the TCR binding to antigen presented on MHC molecules (see Fig. 18) and by interactions between cell molecules on the membrane of T cells and their partners (ligands) on the antigen-presenting cell. Many of these molecules belong to the immunoglobulin superfamily. Some (e.g. CD28 on the T cell and CD80 or CD86 on the antigen-presenting cell) increase the activation of the T cell (see also Fig. 12). Others, e.g. CTLA4 and PD1 on the T cell, and their ligands on the antigen-presenting cell inhibit T-cell activation, and act to limit or switch off the immune response. Several viruses seem to be able to increase expression of these negative regulators in order to escape being killed by the immune system.

Poly-Ig receptor A molecule found on some epithelial cells that helps to transport antibody into secretions such as mucus. Many other molecules contain the characteristic immunoglobulin superfamily domain structure, including some Fc receptors, adhesion molecules (see below) and receptors for growth factors and cytokines. The common feature seems to be an involvement in cell–cell interactions, with the 'breakaway' immunoglobulin molecule the exception rather than the rule.

Killer inhibitory receptors (KIR) Immunoglobulin-family receptors are found on NK cells (see Fig. 15). They recognize MHC molecules on target cells and send negative signals to NK cells that inhibit their activation, and hence prevent killing of targets. NK cells are therefore active only against cells that have lost MHC expression, either as a result of infection (e.g. by viruses) or as a result of malignant transformation (i.e. cancer cells). Some NK cells also express other negative receptors that belong to a different structural family of molecules known as C-lectins. An inhibitory signalling motif (known as an immunoreceptor tyrosine-based inhibitory motif, ITIM) on KIR cytoplasmic tails has an important role in the signal transduction process.

Adhesion molecules A large range of surface molecules help to hold cells together and facilitate cell–cell interactions or binding to blood vessel walls. Many of these are involved in regulating inflammation (see Fig. 7) and attempts to block them for therapeutic purposes are being actively explored. Some of these, as shown in the figure, belong to the immunoglobulin superfamily, and they usually bind to one or a small number of corresponding 'ligands'. Some examples of pairs of molecules important in adhesion are shown in the table. Many of these molecules have both 'common' names and CD numbers (see Appendix III).

Adhesion	Ligand	Type of interaction
CD2	CD58 (LFA3)	T cell–antigen-presenting cell
VCAM-1	VLA-4	Leucocyte–endothelium Leucocyte–leucocyte
ICAM-1 (CD54)		Leucocyte–endothelium
ICAM-2 (CD102) }	LFA-1	T cell–antigen-presenting cell
ICAM-3 (CD50)		
P-selectin E-selectin L-selectin	Vascular addressins, mucin-like molecules (CD34, MadCAM-1, GlyCAM-1)	Leucocyte–endothelium

ICAM, intercellular adhesion molecule; VCAM, vascular cell adhesion molecule.

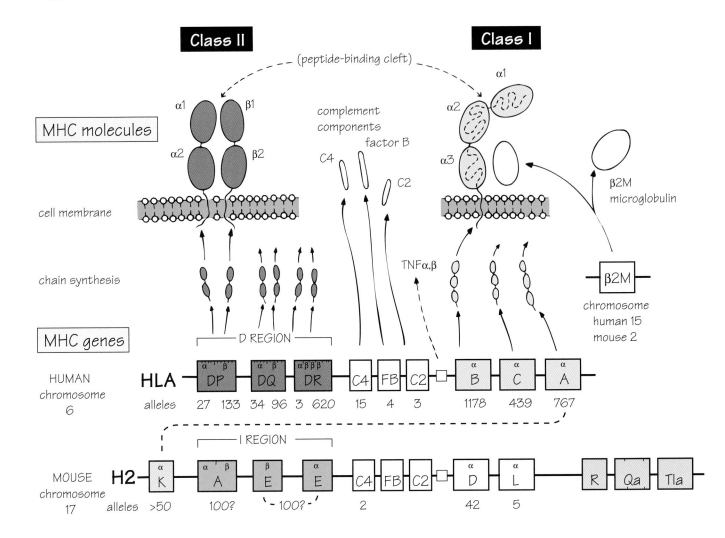

This large and important set of genes owes its rather clumsy-sounding name to the fact that the proteins it codes for were first detected by their effect on transplant rejection, i.e. tissue *incompatibility*. However, it is now clear that their real purpose is to act as receptors binding and stabilizing fragments of antigen and displaying them at the cell surface for T lymphocytes to recognize, via their own receptors, and activate their adaptive immunological functions.

Again, for historical reasons, the MHC in the mouse (extreme bottom line in the figure) is known as **H2**, while in humans it is called **HLA** (human leucocyte antigen). In fact the basic layout of the MHC genes is remarkably similar in all animals so far studied, consisting of a set of class I (shaded in the figure) and a set of class II genes, differing slightly in structure and in the way they interact with T cells (see Fig. 12). In the figure the names of genes are shown

boxed, while the numbers below indicate the approximate number of alternative versions or **alleles** that can occur at each locus. Perhaps the most striking feature of the MHC is the number of different variants that exist in the human population. The number of possible combinations on a single chromosome probably exceeds 3×10^6, so that an individual, with a set of MHC molecules coded for by both chromosomes, can have any one of about 10^{13} combinations, which is part of the problem in transplanting kidneys, etc. (see Fig. 39).

Since HLA typing became a routine procedure, it has emerged that many diseases are significantly more common, or sometimes rarer, in people of a particular HLA type. There are several mechanisms that might account for this but none of them has yet been established to everybody's satisfaction.

Peptide-binding cleft The classic MHC I and II molecules contain a peptide-binding site at the distal end of the molecule from the membrane, formed by two protein α-helices, lying on top of a β-pleated sheet. The binding site, or *groove* as it is often known, can accommodate a peptide of about 9–10 amino acids in length, although for class II MHC molecules, the ends of the groove are open allowing longer peptides to extend out of either end. A wide variety of different peptides can be bound tightly, by interaction between conserved residues in the MHC molecules and the amino acid backbone of the antigen peptide. In order to accommodate the side-chains of the larger amino acids, however, the floor of the groove contains a number of pockets. It is the size and position of these pockets that limit the range of peptides that can be accommodated, focusing the immune response onto only a few defined epitopes.

H2 The MHC of the mouse, carried on chromosome 17. There are at least 20 other minor histocompatibility genes on other chromosomes, numbered H1, H3, H4, etc. but H2 is by far the strongest in causing transplant rejection and the only one known to be involved in normal cell interactions.

HLA The human MHC, on chromosome 6, closely analogous to H2 except that the class I genes lie together and there are three class II genes.

Class I region Class I MHC molecules load peptides derived from the cell cytoplasm (see Fig. 18) and have probably evolved to activate cytotoxic T cells against viruses infecting the cell.

A, B, C The classic human class I genes that present processed peptide antigens to the antigen receptor of CD8 T cells. A is the homologue of K in the mouse.

K, D, L The class I genes of H2, coding for the α chain (MW 44 000), which in combination with β₂-microglobulin (see below) makes up the four-domain K, D and L molecules or 'antigens'.

β2M β₂-Microglobulin (MW 12 000), coded quite separately from the MHC, nevertheless forms part of all class I molecules, stabilizing them on the cell surface. In the mouse there are two allelic forms, but in general β2M is one of the most remarkably conserved molecules known. It is also found free in the serum.

Class IB genes Both human and mouse MHC loci encode a large number (around 50) of genes that code for proteins with a class I-like structure, known as class IB genes. These include Qa and Tla in the mouse, and E, F, G, H, J and X in the human. The function of many of these remains unknown, but some may play a part in controlling innate immunity, perhaps by regulating NK cell activation. Some class IB genes lie outside the MHC locus. One such is the **CD1** family that is specialized for binding glycolipids, especially from mycobacteria, and presenting them to some types of T cells and NK cells.

Class II region As well as the classic class II genes involved in antigen presentation (see below), the class II regions of both mouse and human genome contain genes encoding a number of other molecules involved in the antigen processing pathway (see Fig. 18). These include DM and DO (H2-O and H2-M in the mouse), class II MIIC-like molecules that regulate the loading of peptide fragments onto DP, DQ and DR. The region also contains the LMP genes and the TAP genes (see Fig. 18).

A, E The classic class II genes of H2, which present processed peptide antigen to the antigen receptor of CD4 T cells (see Figs 18, 19 and 21). A and E contain separate genes for the α (MW 33 000) and β (MW 28 000) chains of the four-domain molecule. Unlike class I, class II molecules are expressed only on a minority of cells, namely those that CD4 T cells need to interact with and regulate (see Fig. 12).

DP, DQ, DR The classic human class II genes, which present processed peptide antigens to the antigen receptor of CD4 T cells. The distribution of these different class II molecules within the body is slightly different, but it is still unclear whether each one has a distinct role in the regulation of T-cell responses.

Polymorphism The classic MHC genes in both human and mouse exist in many different alternative (allelic) variants, making these genes the most polymorphic known. The differences between allelic forms lie mostly within or close to the peptide-binding groove, and result in the different alleles binding to different peptide fragments from a particular protein antigen. However, there is also a great deal of polymorphism in the promoter regions of class II MHC, suggesting that the levels of MHC expressed at the cell surface may also be very important. Because MHC molecules are expressed codominantly (i.e. each cell expresses both paternally and maternally inherited alleles), this increases the number of antigens from each pathogen that can be presented to the immune system, and hence makes the immune response more vigorous. Some HLA alleles (e.g. A1 and B8) tend to 'stay together' instead of segregating normally. This is called 'linkage disequilibrium' and may imply that such combinations are of survival value. For example, some HLA alleles have been shown to be linked with a more effective control of HIV, and a slower development of AIDS (see Fig. 28). Not all species show equally great MHC polymorphism: the Syrian hamster, for example, shows little class I variation, perhaps reflecting its isolated lifestyle and hence decreased susceptibility to viral epidemics.

C2, C4, FB Surprisingly, a large number of genes that are structurally unrelated to the classic MHC genes are coded for within the MHC locus. These 'class III' genes include several with immunological function such as complement components involved in the activation of C3, and members of the TNF cytokine family important in inflammation. Although they are less polymorphic than the MHC class I and II genes, some of the genetic association between diseases and the MHC locus may be explained by genetic variation of these class III genes.

HLA-associated diseases (see also Fig. 47). Many diseases show genetic associations with particular HLA alleles. The most remarkable example is the rare sleep abnormality narcolepsy, which virtually only occurs in people carrying the DR2 antigen; the reason is quite unknown. After this, the most striking example is the group of arthropathies involving the sacroiliac joint (ankylosing spondylitis, Reiter's disease, etc.) where one HLA allele (B27) is found in up to 95% of cases, nearly 20 times its frequency in the general population. But numerous other diseases, including almost all of the autoimmune diseases, show a statistically significant association with particular HLA antigens or groups of antigens, especially in the class II region. The explanation probably lies in the ability or otherwise of the HLA molecule to present particular microbial peptides or, alternatively, self-antigens.

12 The T-cell receptor

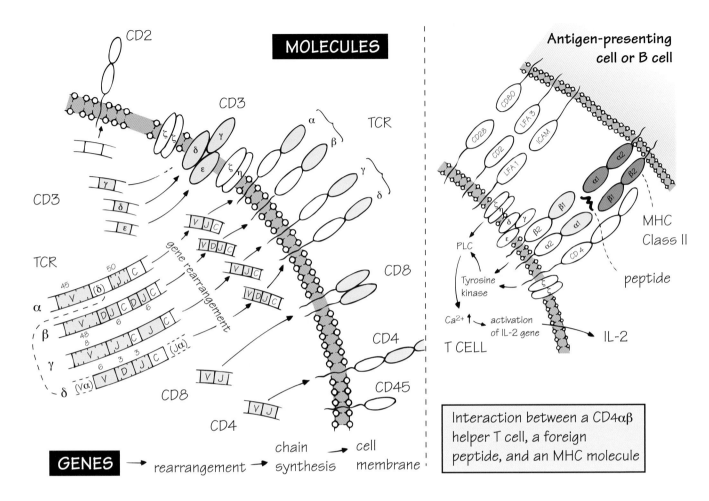

MOLECULES

Antigen-presenting cell or B cell

Interaction between a CD4αβ helper T cell, a foreign peptide, and an MHC molecule

GENES → rearrangement → chain synthesis → cell membrane

It had been evident for many years that T lymphocytes have a surface receptor for antigen, with roughly similar properties to the antibody on B lymphocytes, but furious controversy raged as to whether the two molecules were in fact identical. The T-cell receptor (TCR) was finally identified unambiguously in 1983–4 by the use of monoclonal antibodies to study the fine structure of the molecule and use of DNA probing to identify the corresponding genes.

The TCR has the typical domain structure of an immunoglobulin-family molecule. Its three-dimensional structure is rather similar to that of one arm of an antibody molecule (see Fig. 14), and is made up of two major chains (α, β) each of two domains. A second (γδ) combination is found on some T cells instead of αβ. However, instead of interacting directly with intact macromolecules as does antibody, the TCR recognizes very short stretches of peptide antigen bound to an MHC molecule (as illustrated in the right-hand part of the figure for a T cell of the helper variety). The α and β chains associate on the cell membrane with other transmembrane proteins to form the CD3 complex. This complex, in association with other molecules (e.g. CD4, CD8), is responsible for transducing an activation signal into the T cell.

An unusual feature of the αβ chains of the TCR, which is shared with the heavy and light chain of the antibody molecule, is that the genes for different parts of each polypeptide chain do not lie together on the chromosome, so that unwanted segments of DNA, and subsequently of RNA, have to be excised to bring them together. This process is known as **gene rearrangement** and occurs only in T and B cells, so that in all other cells the genes remain in their non-functional 'germline' configuration. Once this rearrangement has occurred in an individual lymphocyte, that cell is committed to a unique receptor, and therefore a unique antigen-recognizing ability. In this and the following figure, the portions of genes and proteins that are coloured blue are those thought to have evolved from the primitive V region, although they do not all show the same degree of variability.

TCR The T-cell receptor. It is made up of one α (MW 50 000) and one β (MW 45 000) chain, each with an outer variable domain, an inner constant domain and short intramembrane and cytoplasmic regions. Some T cells, especially early in fetal life and in some organs such as the gut and skin, express the alternative γδ receptor and seem to recognize a different set of antigens including some bacterial gly-colipids. γδ T cells are rare in humans, but are a major proportion of T cells in other animals including cows, pigs and sheep. The way in which individual T cells are first positively and then negatively **selected** in the thymus to ensure they only recognize self-MHC plus a foreign peptide is described in Fig. 16.

CD3 A complex of three chains, γ (MW 25 000), δ (MW 20 000) and ε (MW 20 000), essential to all T-cell function. Also associated with the TCR–CD3 complex are two other signalling molecules, ζ and η. All these molecules contain sequences known as immunoreceptor tyrosine-based activation motifs (ITAMs), which allow them to bind to phosphorylating enzymes in the cell and hence lead to **T-cell activation**. Interaction of antigen (i.e. MHC plus peptide) with this whole complex causes many TCR complexes to cluster together on the surface of the cell, forming an 'immunological synapse'.

CD4 A single-chain molecule (MW 60 000) found on human helper T cells. It interacts with MHC class II molecules (as shown in the figure), and is therefore recruited into the vicinity of the TCR, bringing with it a T-cell-specific kinase, lck, which binds to its cytoplasmic portion and which facilitates the process of T-cell activation. CD4 is also the major receptor which HIV uses to enter the T cell (see Fig. 28).

CD8 A molecule (MW 75 000) found on most cytotoxic T cells. In humans it is composed of two identical chains, but the equivalent in the mouse has two different chains (Ly2/3). It is involved in interacting with MHC class I molecules. Because of their close association with the TCR, CD4 and CD8 are sometimes known as 'coreceptors'.

Costimulation Binding of the TCR to the MHC–peptide antigen is not, by itself, sufficient to activate T cells efficiently. T cells need simultaneously to receive signals via other cell-surface receptors, which bind ligands on the antigen-presenting cell. Two examples of such 'costimulatory' interactions are those between CD2 on the T cell and LFA-3 (CD58) on the antigen-presenting cell, and between CD28 on the T cell and CD80 (B7.1) or CD86 (B7.2) on the antigen-presenting cell. This is often called the 'two-signal' model of T-cell activation (although in reality there are many more than two signals involved). It has important implications for the induction of tolerance (see Fig. 22) because when T cells recognize antigen in the absence of the right costimulation they can become unresponsive to future encounters with antigen (such T cells are described as **tolerant**, or sometimes **anergic**). Other costimulatory molecules (e.g. CTLA-4 and PD1 on the T cell which interact with their respective ligands on the antigen-presenting cells) transmit negative signals that are important to prevent over-activation of T cells. Blocking these negative interactions is showing promising results as a way of improving immune responses to chronic viral infections (see Fig. 27) and cancer (see Fig. 42).

CD45 This transmembrane protein was originally known as 'leuco-cyte common antigen' because it is found on all white blood cells. However, on T cells it distinguishes 'memory' T cells (those that have already encountered antigen) from 'naive' T cells (those that have yet to encounter antigens). The extracellular portion of CD45 exists in a number of variant forms. The shortest form (known as CD45Ro) is found on activated and memory T cells, but not on most naive T cells (see Fig. 15). In contrast, one of the longer forms (CD45RA) is found predominantly on naive T cells. The intracellular portion codes for a tyrosine phosphatase, which plays a key part in TCR regulation via regulation of the tyrosine kinase lck (see above).

Gene rearrangement The TCR genes contain up to 100 V genes and numerous J and D genes, so that to make a single chain, one of each must be linked up to the correct C gene. This is done by excision of intervening DNA sequences and further excision in the mRNA, even-tually producing a single V–D–J–C RNA to code for the polypeptide chain. When all the possible combinations of α and β chains are taken into account, the number of different TCR molecules available to an individual may be as high as 10^{15} (see also Fig. 10).

Antigen Shown in the figure as a short peptide, in this case bound by an MHC molecule and then recognized by the TCR (for details see Fig. 18). The strength of interaction between one TCR and one MHC–peptide complex is relatively weak, but the combined effect of many simultaneous interactions on the T cell, aided by CD4–MHC or CD8–MHC interactions, results in T-cell activation. Interestingly, some antigen peptides (antagonist peptides) can have the opposite effect, in that they somehow turn off T-cell activation and make the T cells unresponsive to further stimulation. Such peptides might have possible therapeutic uses in regulating unwanted immune reactions such as allergies or autoimmunity.

T-cell activation ultimately results in the transcription of several hundred genes that determine T-cell proliferation, differentiation and effector function. A key early event is the movement of many TCR molecules on the surface of the T cell into the contact area between the T cell and the antigen-presenting cell (the immunological synapse). This increased local concentration leads to tyrosine phosphorylation of **ITAMs** on the cytoplasmic tails of several of the CD3 chains. This in turn recruits further tyrosine kinases (e.g. zap) and ultimately leads to activation of transcription factors, proteins that bind specific sites on DNA and hence regulate transcription of particular sets of genes. One key step in T cells is the activation of the transcription factor NF-AT, and it is this step that is inhibited by cyclosporine and FK506, important immunosuppressants used clinically to block transplant rejection (see Fig. 39).

IL-2 One of the main events that follows recognition of antigen by T cells is that the responding T cells undergo several rounds of cell divi-sion (a phenomenon known as clonal expansion). T-cell proliferation is driven largely by secretion from the T cells themselves of the cytokine interleukin 2 (IL-2). IL-2 was one of the first of the family of **cytokines** to be identified. As well as its major role in inducing T-cell proliferation, it has effects on B lymphocytes, macrophages, eosinophils, etc. (see Fig. 24). T-cell activation also results in secretion of many other cytokines (see Figs 21, 23 and 24).

Superantigens There is one exception to the very high specificity of T cell–peptide–MHC interactions: certain molecules, e.g. some viruses and staphylococcal enterotoxins, have the curious ability to bind to both MHC class II and the TCR β chain *outside* the peptide-binding site. The result is that a whole 'family' of T cells respond, rather than a single clone, with excessive and potentially damaging over-production of cytokines.

13 Antibody diversification and synthesis

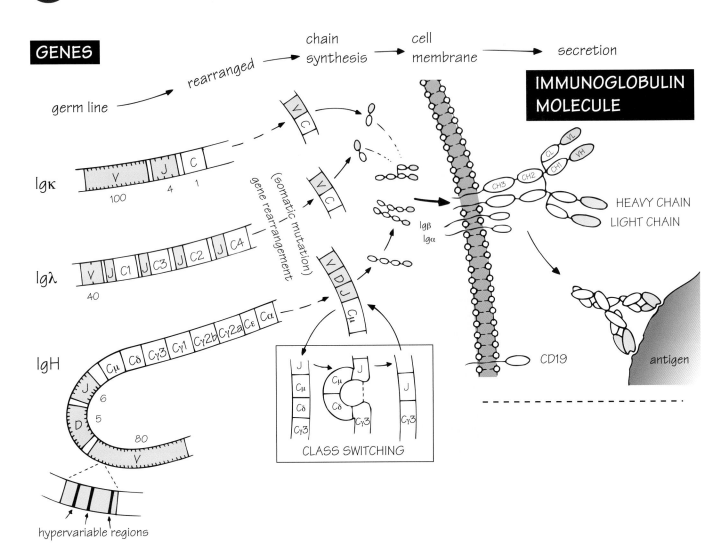

In contrast to the MHC and the T-cell receptor, the existence of the antibody, or **immunoglobulin** (Ig), molecule has been known for over 100 years and its basic structure for about 50, which makes it one of the most studied and best understood molecules in biology.

The two-chain multidomain structure characteristic of MHC and T-cell receptors is seen here in a slightly more complex form, a typical Ig molecule being made up of four chains: a pair of **heavy** chains and a pair of **light** chains (for structural details see Fig. 14). Two main kinds of diversity are found within these chains: in the **constant** regions of the heavy chains are the variations that classify Ig molecules into classes and subclasses with different biological effects, while the much more extensive variations in the **variable** regions (blue in the figure) are responsible for the shape of the antigen-binding site and thus of the antigen specificity of the Ig molecule.

Within B lymphocytes, the genes for Ig heavy and light chains are put together by a process of rearrangement at the DNA level followed by further excisions in the mRNA, very much as in T cells with their receptor, one important difference being that in B, but not T, cells, further **somatic mutation** in the variable regions can occur. Finally, the polypeptide chains are synthesized on ribosomes, similar to other proteins, assembled and exported – some to reside on the cell surface as receptors and others to be secreted into the blood as **antibody**.

Ig Immunoglobulin; the name given to all globulins with antibody activity. It has replaced the old term 'gamma globulin' because not all antibodies have gamma electrophoretic mobility.

Igκ, Igλ, IgH Three genetic loci on different chromosomes (see Fig. 47), which code for the light chain (κ, λ) and heavy (H) chain of the Ig molecule. A typical Ig molecule has two H chains and two L chains, either both κ or both λ.

Germline This denotes those genes in the ova and sperm giving rise to successive generations, which can be regarded as a continuous family tree stretching back to the earliest forms of life. Mutations and other genetic changes in these genes are passed to subsequent generations and are what natural selection works on. Changes that occur in any other cells of the body are 'somatic' and affect only the individual, being lost when death occurs. This includes the changes in the DNA of B lymphocytes that lead to the formation of the Ig molecule. The antibody germline genes have presumably been selected as indispensable, and many of them have been shown to code for antibodies against common bacteria, confirming that bacterial infection was probably the main stimulus for the evolution of antibody.

V Variable region genes. Their number ranges from two (mouse λ chain) to about 350 (mouse κ chain; the numbers shown in the figure are for the human). The greatest variation is found in three short **hypervariable** regions, which code for the amino acids that form the combining site and make contact with the antigen. V genes are classified into **families** on the basis of overall sequence similarity.

C Constant region genes. In the light chains, these code for a single domain only, but in the heavy chains there are three or four domains, numbered CH 1, 2, 3, (4). Which of the eight (mouse) or nine (human) C genes is in use by a particular B lymphocyte determines the class and subclass of the resulting Ig molecule (IgM, IgG, etc.; see Fig. 14).

J Joining region genes, coding for the short J segment. Note that in the κ and H chains, the different J genes lie together while in the λ chain each C gene has its own. In primitive vertebrates there are repeated V–J–C segments, which restricts the number of possible combinations.

D region genes are found only on IgH, where they provide additional possibilities for hypervariability.

Gene rearrangement occurs in the Ig genes of B lymphocytes in a similar way to the TCR genes of T lymphocytes. First, the intervening segments of DNA ('introns') between the V and J (and D if present) genes are excised in such a way as to bring together one particular V and one J gene. The excision and joining is an imprecise process, generating even more diversity, but also resulting in many B cells failing to produce a proper Ig molecule, and therefore dying during development. Once a correctly formed Ig molecule has been produced by rearrangement on one chromosome, the Ig locus on the other chromosome is switched off ('allelic exclusion'), thus ensuring a B cell only ever expresses antibody of one specificity. This unique process of DNA rearrangements is catalysed by a complex of enzymes, many of which are involved in DNA repair functions in other cells. However, the first cleavage of DNA that initiates the recombination event is catalysed by two specialized enzymes, RAG-1 and RAG-2 (recombination activating genes). These enzymes are expressed only in developing B and T cells, and knocking out these genes in mice results in a complete absence of B or T cells.

Class switching can occur within the individual B cell by further excisions of DNA, which allow the same VDJ segment to lie next to a different C gene, leading to antibodies with the same specificity for antigen but a different constant region (see Fig. 14). This allows the same antigen to be subjected to various different forms of attack. The decision which class or subclass to switch to is largely regulated by cytokines released locally by helper T cells; thus, IL-4 favours IgE, IL-5 IgA, IFNγ IgG3, etc. (these examples are from the mouse).

Somatic mutation After they have been activated by antigen and T cells, B cells migrate into the **germinal centres** (see Fig. 19). Here they undergo extensive rounds of replication. In addition, individual B cells introduce point mutations into their immunoglobulin genes, a process known as somatic hypermutation, which requires cytidine deaminase, an enzyme that chemically modifies individual bases on the DNA. After mutation, the B cells with the highest affinity are selected to survive, and become part of the **memory** lymphocyte populations. In this way, successive exposures to antigen select for ever higher affinity antibodies, a process known as affinity maturation.

CD19 One of the molecules (the complement receptor CR2 is another) that need to be bound in order to fully activate the B cell, thus playing a 'coreceptor' role somewhat analogous to CD4, CD8 and CD28 on the T cell. CD19 is also a convenient 'marker' for B cells, because it is not expressed on other types of cell.

Origins of diversity Four features of antibody contribute to the enormous number of possible antigen-binding sites and thus of antibody specificities: (i) gene rearrangement allows any V, D and J genes to become associated; (ii) a heavy chain can pair with either a κ or λ light chain; (iii) V–D and D–J joining is imprecise, allowing the addition or removal of a few DNA bases; and (iv) mutations are introduced into the V genes of an individual B cell after antigen stimulation (this would be a case of **somatic mutation**, see above). Because of all these possibilities it is difficult to put a number on the size of the Ig repertoire, but it may be as high as 10^{10}. Note that diversity within the MHC is generated in a quite different way, individuals having only one or two of the allelic variants of each gene. The members of a species differ from each other much more in their MHC genes and molecules than in their Ig and T-cell receptors, of which they all have a fairly complete set with only minor inherited differences.

Igα, Igβ Two molecules that form a link between cell-surface Ig and intracellular signalling pathways, analogous to CD3 on the T cell.

14 Antibody structure and function

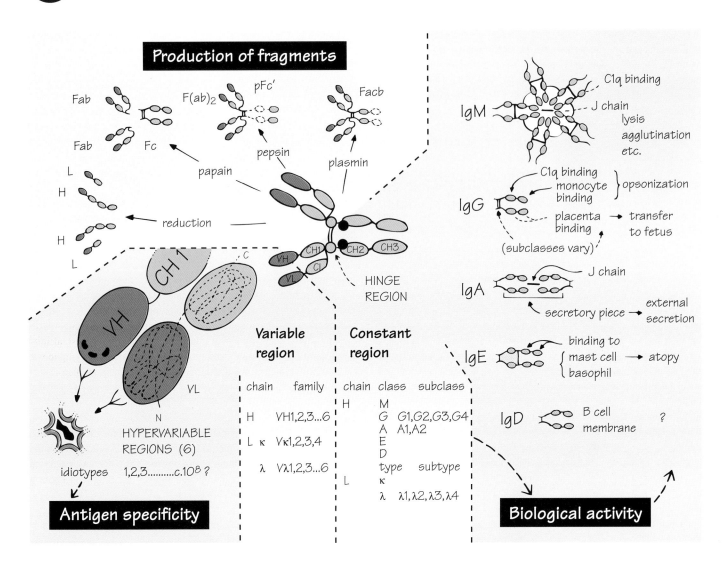

Considering that the antibody in serum is a mixture of perhaps 100 million slightly different types of molecule, the unravelling of its structure was no mean feat. Early work depended on separation into fragments by chemical treatment (top left in figure); the fine details have come from amino acid sequencing and X-ray crystallography, both of which require the use of completely homogeneous (monoclonal) antibody. This was originally available only in the form of myeloma proteins, the product of malignant B lymphocytes, but is produced nowadays by the hybridoma method (see Fig. 15) or by genetic engineering in bacteria, yeast or a variety of mammalian cell types.

A typical antibody molecule (IgG, centre) has 12 domains, arranged in two heavy and two light (H and L) chains, linked through cysteine residues by disulphide bonds so that the domains lie together in pairs, the whole molecule having the shape of a flexible **Y**. In each chain the N-terminal domain is the most **variable**, the rest being relatively **constant**. Within the variable (V) regions, the maximum variation in amino acid sequence is seen in the six **hypervariable** regions (three per chain) which come together to form the **antigen-binding site** (bottom left in figure). The constant (C) regions vary mainly in those portions that

interact with complement or various cell-surface receptors; the right-hand part of the figure shows the different features of the C region in the five **classes** of antibody: M, G, A, E and D. The result is a huge variety of molecules able to bring any antigen into contact with any one of several effective disposal mechanisms. The basic structure (MW about 160 000) can form dimers (IgA, MW 400 000) or pentamers (IgM, MW 900 000) (see right-hand side of figure).

There are species differences, especially in the heavy chain subclasses, which have evolved comparatively recently; the examples shown here illustrate human antibodies. Interestingly, camels and llamas also have antibodies with only heavy chains. These antibodies may be able to attach to some targets not accessible to conventional antibodies, and examples are being tested as possible new ways of preventing infection by viruses such as HIV (see Fig. 28). The carbohydrate side-chains (shown here in black) may constitute up to 12% of the whole molecule.

Note: The illustration shows an IgG molecule with its 12 domains stylized. The actual three-dimensional structure is more like the molecule shown binding to antigen in Fig. 13 (extreme right).

36 *Immunology at a Glance*, Tenth Edition. J.H.L. Playfair and B.M. Chain. © 2013 John Wiley & Sons, Ltd. Published 2013 by John Wiley & Sons, Ltd.

Fragments produced by chemical treatment: these fragments were of great importance in elucidating the chemical structure of antibody. Fab and F(ab)$_2$ fragments allow binding to specific antigen in the absence of secondary interactions with other cells mediated via the constant region.
• H, L: heavy and light chains which, being only disulphide-linked, separate under reducing conditions.
• Fab: antigen-binding fragment (papain digestion).
• Fc: crystallizable (because relatively homogeneous) fragment (papain digestion).
• F(ab)$_2$: two Fab fragments united by disulphide bonds (pepsin digestion).

Affinity and avidity The strength of binding between one V domain and an antigen is called the affinity of the antibody (see Fig. 20). Typically, it is of the order of 10^8 L/mol or above. However, antibody molecules have two, or in the case of IgM 10, identical binding domains. If the antigen recognized also has repeated units, such as the surface of many bacteria or viruses, one antibody molecule can make multiple attachments to the same target antigen. The strength of this overall binding is known as the antibody's avidity. It can be much greater than the affinity, typically 100 times more for a divalent antibody and up to 100 000 times more for IgM.

Chains The heavy and two types of light (κ, λ) chains are coded for by genes on different chromosomes, but sequence homologies suggest that all Ig domains originated from a common 'precursor' molecule about 110 amino acids long (see Fig. 10). A proportion of antibodies consisting only of heavy chains are found in some species (e.g. camels and llamas). These antibodies are narrower and can sometimes fit into sites conventional antibodies cannot reach, which may make them useful for some types of therapy.

Classes Physical, antigenic and functional variations between constant regions define the five main classes of heavy chain: M, G, A, E and D. These are different molecules, all of which are present in all members of most higher species. Points of interest are listed below.

IgM is usually the first class of antibody made in a response and is also thought to have been the first to appear during evolution (see Fig. 46). Because its pentameric structure gives it up to 10 antigen-combining sites, it can show high avidity, even though it may have a relatively low specific affinity. It is therefore extremely efficient at binding and agglutinating microorganisms early in the response. However, it is also very efficient at making larger immune complexes (see Fig. 20), which can activate unwanted inflammation and disease (see Fig 36). Its production is therefore downregulated as soon as sufficient IgG has been generated.

IgG is a later development that owes its value to the ability of its Fc portion to bind avidly to C1q (see Fig. 6) and to receptors on phagocytic cells (see Fig. 9). It also gains access to the extravascular spaces and (via the placenta) to the fetus. In most species, IgG has become further diversified into subclasses (see below).

IgA is the major antibody of secretions such as tears, sweat and the contents of lungs, gut, urine, etc., where, thanks to its secretory piece (see below), it avoids digestion. It blocks the entry of microorganisms from these external surfaces to the tissues themselves.

IgE is a curious molecule whose main property is to bind to mast cells and promote their degranulation. The desirable and undesirable consequences of this are discussed in Fig. 35.

IgD appears to function only on the surface of B cells, where it may have some regulatory role. In the mouse it is unusual in having two instead of three constant regions in the heavy chain.

Subclasses, subtypes Within classes, smaller variations between constant regions define the subclasses found in different molecules of all members of an individual species. The IgG subclasses are generally the most varied. All these variants found in all individuals of a species are called 'isotypic'.

Allotypes In contrast, 'allotypic' variations (not shown in the figure) distinguish the Ig molecules of some individuals from others (compare blood groups). They are genetically determined and occur mainly in the C regions. No biological function has yet been discovered. Unlike blood groups, Ig allotypes are expressed singly on individual B cells, a process known as 'allelic exclusion', which shows that only one of the cell's two sets of chromosomes are used for making antibody – presumably the first one to rearrange its Ig genes successfully.

Hypervariable regions Three parts of each of the variable regions of heavy and light chains, spaced roughly equally apart in the amino acid sequence (see lower left of figure) but brought close together as the chain folds into a β-pleated sheet, form the antigen-combining site. It is because of the enormous degree of variation in the DNA coding for these regions that the total number of combinations is so high. The hypervariable regions are also unusually susceptible to further **somatic mutation**, which occurs during B-cell proliferation within the germinal centre of lymph nodes or spleen. This further increases the range of available combining sites.

Idiotypes In many cases, antibody molecules with different antigen-combining sites can in turn be distinguished by other antibodies made against them. The latter are known as 'anti-idiotypic', implying that each combining site is associated with a different shape, although this is not always the antigen-binding site itself. Anti-idiotypic antibodies are thought to be formed normally and may possibly help to regulate immune responses.

Hinge region Both flexibility and proteolytic digestion are facilitated by the repeated proline residues in this part of the molecule. In IgM, the hinge region is as large as a normal domain, and is called CH2, so that the other two constant region domains are called CH3 and CH4.

J chain A glycopeptide molecule that aids polymerization of IgA and IgM.

Secretory piece A polypeptide derived from the poly-Ig receptor (see Fig. 10) and added to IgA dimers in epithelial cells to enable them to be transported across the epithelium and secreted into the gut, tears, milk, etc. where IgA predominates.

C1q The first component of the classic complement sequence, a hexavalent glycoprotein activated by binding to CH2 domains of IgM and some IgG subclasses (in the human, IgG1 and IgG3; see Fig. 6).

Antibodies for therapy Pure preparations of monoclonal antibodies are increasingly in clinical use, notably for autoimmune diseases and cancer (see Figs 38 and 42). Various strategies are available to avoid the recipient mounting an immune response against these antibodies, including the use of 'humanized' mouse monoclonals or of human cells genetically engineered to produce antibodies of the desired specificity.

15 Lymphocytes

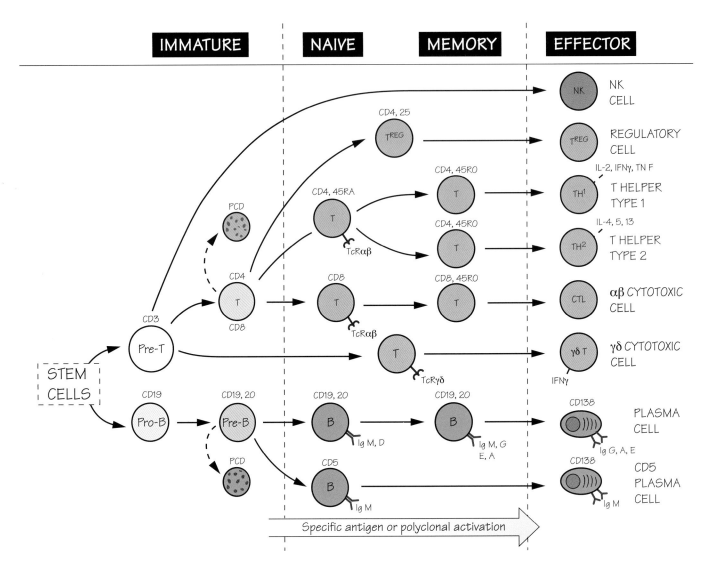

As befits the cell of adaptive immunity, the lymphocyte has several unique features: restricted receptors permitting each cell to respond to an individual antigen (the basis of **specificity**), clonal proliferation and long lifespan (the basis of **memory**), and recirculation from the tissues back into the bloodstream, which ensures that specific memory following a local response has a body-wide **distribution**.

The discovery in the early 1960s of the two major lymphocyte sub-populations, **T** (thymus-dependent; top) and **B** (bursa or bone marrow-dependent; bottom), had roughly the same impact on cellular immunology as the double helix on molecular biology. The first property of T cells to be distinguished was that of 'helping' B cells to make antibody, but further subdivisions have subsequently come to light, based on both functional and physical differences (top right). In the figure, the main surface features (or 'markers') of the various stages of lymphocyte differentiation are given, using mainly the CD classification (see Appendix III) but also indicating the production of key cytokines.

Cells resembling lymphocytes, but without characteristic T-cell or B-cell markers, are referred to as 'null'. This group probably includes early T cells, B cells and 'natural killer' cells important in tumour and virus immunity. In blood and lymphoid organs, up to 10% of lymphocytes are 'null'.

One of the most exciting developments in biology was the discovery that it is possible to perpetuate individual lymphocytes by fusing them with a tumour cell. In the case of B lymphocytes, this can mean an endless supply of individual, or **monoclonal**, antibodies, which has had far-reaching applications in the diagnosis and treatment of disease and the study of cell surfaces. Indeed, the classification of lymphocytes themselves, and of most other cells too, is now mainly based on patterns of reactivity with a large range of monoclonal typing antibodies (see Appendix III).

In the case of T cells, it is also possible to keep them proliferating indefinitely in culture by judicious application of their specific antigen and non-specific growth factors such as IL-2 (see Figs 23 and 24). The properties of the resulting **lines** or **clones** have given much information on the regulation of normal T-cell function.

Naïve cells Once mature, lymphocytes (B or T) circulate through blood and lymph nodes in search of specific antigen. These cells can be very long-lived, and divide only very rarely. Such lymphocytes, which have yet to encounter antigen, are known as **naïve** or virgin (see Fig. 17). Naïve T cells enter lymph nodes from blood at special sites known as high endothelial venules (HEV). They then travel though the lymph node in search of antigen presented on the surface of antigen-presenting dendritic cells in the T-cell areas of lymphoid tissues.

Memory cells After lymphocytes encounter antigen they enter cell division, in order to increase the number of cells specific for that particular antigen. A proportion of cells then become memory cells. The migratory paths of memory cells and **naïve** cells are quite distinct; memory cells leave blood vessels at the site of an infection, enter tissues and then travel back to lymph nodes via the lymphatics. **Memory** cells can persist for many years, dividing every few months, even in the absence of further antigen stimulation. Most memory T cells are conveniently distinguished from naïve T cells by expression of the CD45RO and CD45RA surface markers, respectively.

Effector cells After they encounter antigen, a proportion of lymphocytes differentiate into effector cells, expressing molecules required to perform their ultimate function in defending the body against disease. B-cell effectors mostly settle in the bone marrow, where they produce antibody, and are known as **plasma cells**. T cells can become **helper cells** (T^H), **cytotoxic cells** (CTLs, T^C) or **regulatory cells** (T^{REG}). Effector T cells migrate to the site of infection, and usually stop recirculating or dividing further.

NK Natural killer cells are cytotoxic to some virus-infected cells and some tumours (see also Fig. 42). NK cells express a special class of polymorphic **killer inhibitory receptors** (KIRs) which bind self-MHC and then negatively signal to the cell to prevent activation of cytotoxicity. NK cells are therefore only activated when cells lose expression of MHC molecules, such as sometimes occurs during viral infection or tumour growth. They thus form an important counterpart to **cytotoxic T cells** (see below), which kill cells only when they *do* express MHC molecules. An intermediate cell type known as the NK-T cell uses a restricted set of T-cell receptors to respond to bacterial glycolipids presented by CD1 molecules, but has many of the properties of NK cells.

T cells The subset of lymphocytes that develop within the thymus (see Fig. 16). All T cells express one form of the **TCR** with which they recognize antigen.

Two alternative types of TCR exist, consisting either of a dimer made up of an α and a β chain or, a γδ dimer (see Fig. 12).

CD A classification of the molecules found on the surface of haemo-poietic cells based on reaction with panels of monoclonal antibodies. The profile of CD antigens expressed by cells is used to classify them. A list of CD numbers is given in Appendix III, but it should be noted that some older functional names (C3 receptor, Fc receptor, etc.) are still in use.

Polyclonal activation Stimulation of many clones, rather than the few or single clones normally stimulated by an antigen. Because the first sign of activation is often mitosis, polyclonal activators are sometimes known as 'mitogens'. Several T-cell polyclonal activators are of plant origin, e.g. concanavalin A (CON A) and phytohaemagglutinin (PHA). Dextran sulphate, lipopolysaccharide (e.g. *Salmonella* endotoxin) and *Staphylococcus aureus* cell wall are normally mitogenic only for B

cells. They have provided a useful tool for the study of lymphocyte activation.

Cytotoxic T cell (T^C) Cytotoxic T cells kill cells expressing their specific antigen target. The killing is triggered by binding of the **TCR** to MHC bound to appropriate antigen peptide fragments (see Fig. 18). The target cell is killed either by the release of perforin and granzymes, or by expression of CD154 (also known as Fas ligand) on the T-cell surface that engages CD95 (Fas) on the target. In both cases, the target cell dies by **programmed cell death** (also known as apoptosis). **CTLs** are key cells in virus immunity (see Figs 27 and 28) and immune responses to tumours (Fig. 42). Prolonged stimulation of cytotoxic T cells, e.g. due to chronic infection or cancer, can lead to cell exhaustion, in which large numbers of T cells persist but have greatly impaired cytotoxic activity and cytokine production.

Helper T cell (T^H) The CD4 T cell is essential for most antibody and cell-mediated responses (see Figs 18, 19 and 21). CD4 T cells can be further subdivided on the basis of which cytokines they secrete. T^{H1} cells, for example, make cytokines such as IFNγ and TNF-α important for activating macrophages or **delayed hypersensitivity**. In contrast, T^{H2} cells make cytokines needed for helping B cells to make certain types of antibody, especially IgE. The most recent T-helper subtype to be defined are confusingly named T^{H17} because they secrete the cytokine IL-17. These cells are important in recruiting neutrophils, and especially in protection against fungal infection (see Fig. 30), but they are also frequently associated with autoimmunity (see Fig. 38).

Regulatory T cell (T^{REG}) These cells are the major regulators of the immune response. They can be distinguished from other T cells by the expression of high levels of CD25 and the transcription factor FOXP3. "Natural" T^{REG} come directly from the thymus, and help maintain self-tolerance (Fig. 22). Other types of T^{REG} can be induced during infection and work by the release of inhibitory cytokines such as IL-10 and TGF-β.

B cells Lymphocytes whose antigen-specific receptor is antibody (Ig, see Figs 13 and 14). B cells develop in the bone marrow (or liver in the fetus) where they pass through various stages (pre-B and pro-B cells) that are required for the full assembly of the antibody molecule (see Fig. 13). Many cells die during this developmental process due to incorrect antibody assembly or because they recognize self-antigen B cells produce.

Plasma cells are non-motile and are found predominantly in bone marrow or spleen. Their cytoplasm is completely filled with an enormously enlarged rough endoplasmic reticulum devoted to synthesis and secretion of soluble antibody. Most plasma cells are short-lived (1–2 weeks) but some may survive much longer. Some antibody formation, especially IgM, does not require T-cell help, and is called 'thymus independent'. It usually involves direct cross-linking of antibody on the B-cell surface by multivalent antigens such as bacterial cell wall polysaccharides. T-independent responses tend to be short-lived and show very weak memory.

PCD Programmed cell death, also known as *apoptosis*; a process by which cells are induced to die without damage to surrounding tissue. A very high proportion of both B and T cells die in this way because they fail to rearrange their receptor genes properly, or because they threaten to be 'self-reactive' (see Fig. 38). Mutations in CD95, a key receptor activating PCD in lymphocytes, are associated with a multi organ autoimmune disease, illustrating the importance of this pathway in regulating the normal immune response.

16 Primary lymphoid organs and lymphopoiesis

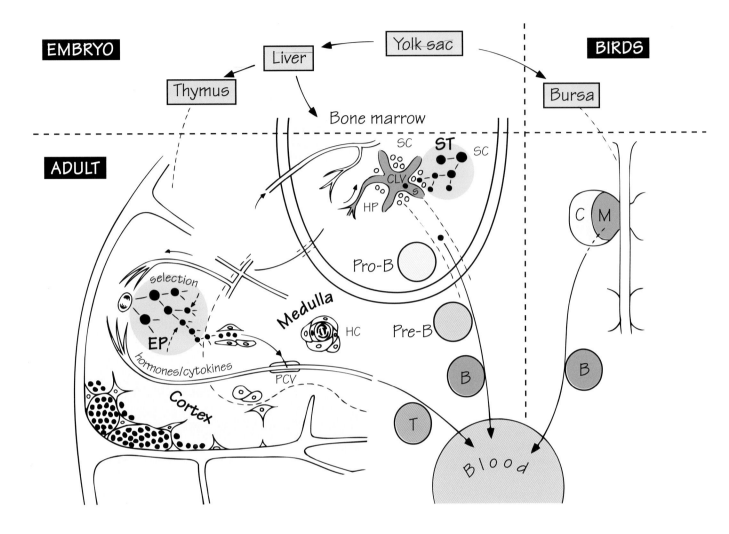

The first strong evidence for distinct lymphocyte populations was the complementary effects in birds of early removal of the **thymus** (which mainly affects cell-mediated immunity) and the **bursa of Fabricius** (which affects antibody responses). A continuing puzzle has been the identification of what represents the bursa in mammals; despite a phase when 'gut-associated lymphoid tissue' was a popular candidate, current opinion considers there to be no true analogue, the liver taking over the function of B-cell maturation in the fetus, the bone marrow in the adult.

The production of both B and T lymphocytes is a highly random and, at first glance, wasteful process, quite unlike any other form of haemopoiesis. It involves the rearrangement of genes to give each cell a unique receptor molecule (for details see Figs 12 and 13) and the elimination of all those cells that fail to achieve this, plus those that carry receptors that would recognize 'self' molecules and thus be potentially self-destructive (see Fig. 38). As recognition by T cells is more complex, involving the MHC as well as foreign antigen (see Figs 11, 12 and 18), production of T cells is a correspondingly more elaborate process, requiring two separate selection steps, one **for** self-MHC and one **against** self-antigens.

Both B- and T-cell development involves rapid and extensive cell proliferation. Cytokines (especially IL-2 and IL-7) have a key role in driving this cell expansion, and genetic defects in their receptors (e.g. common γ-chain deficiency) results in profound immunodeficiency (see Fig. 33). The repair of these genetic defects has been one of the first successful applications of the novel field of gene therapy to medicine.

Yolk sac

The source of the earliest haemopoietic tissue, including the lymphocyte precursors.

Bursa

In birds, B lymphocytes differentiate in the bursa of Fabricius, a cloacal outgrowth with many crypts and follicles, which reaches its maximum size a few weeks after birth and thereafter atrophies. Despite claims for the appendix, tonsil, etc., there is probably no mammalian analogue.

M Medulla; the region where the first stem cells colonize the bursal follicles.

C Cortex; the site of proliferation of the B lymphocytes.

Liver

During fetal life in mammals, the major haemopoietic and lymphopoietic organ.

Bone marrow

SC Haematopoietic stem cells and stem cells of the B-cell lineage.

ST Stromal cells provide the structure and microenvironment in the bone marrow that allow B-cell differentiation.

HP Haemopoietic area. The anatomical location of lymphopoiesis in liver and bone marrow is not exactly known, but it presumably proceeds alongside the other haemopoietic pathways, in close association with macrophages and stromal cells. At least 70% of B cells die before release, probably because of faulty rearrangement of their immunoglobulin genes (see Fig. 13) or excessive self-reactivity.

S Sinus, collecting differentiated cells for discharge into the blood via the central longitudinal vein (**CLV**).

Thymus

A two-lobed organ lying in the upper chest (in birds, in the neck), derived from outgrowths of the third and fourth branchial cleft and pharyngeal pouch. Like the bursa, it is largest in early life, although its subsequent atrophy is slower. In it, bone marrow-derived stem cells are converted into mature T lymphocytes. Remarkably, a second, much smaller thymus has only recently been discovered in the neck of mice. Some of the interpretations of classic thymectomy experiments on immune function may therefore have to be reinterpreted.

Thymocytes Immature T cells found within the thymus. The majority of thymocytes express both CD4 and CD8 on their surface, and are known as 'double positives'. Over 90% of thymocytes die within the thymus before reaching maturity.

EP Epithelial cells within the thymus support thymic development by the production of cytokines and hormones, and by cell-surface interaction with **thymocytes**. Thymic epithelial cells express both class I and class II MHC molecules and have an important role in **selection**. Thymic epithelial cells also have a special mechanism for expressing small amounts of a large number of 'non-thymus' proteins, which contributes to the establishment of self-tolerance (see Fig. 22). Failure of this mechanism in rare genetic diseases leads to generalized autoimmunity and death.

Hormones Numerous soluble factors extracted from the thymus (e.g. thymosins) were shown to stimulate the maturation of T cells, as judged by function or surface markers or both. Although several of these hormones are being tested for their ability to boost immunological function in a whole variety of diseases, their name is probably a misnomer as they are found in many other tissues and are not thought to have an important role in thymic development. The major maturing and differentiating factors are the cytokines (see Fig. 24), deficiencies of which can cause profound defects in lymphocyte development.

Cortex Dark-staining outer part packed with lymphocytes, compartmentalized by elongated epithelial cells. The process of proliferation and selection occurs mainly here.

Medulla Inner, predominantly epithelial part, to which cortical lymphocytes migrate before export via venules and lymphatics. The final stages of selection may occur at the cortico-medullary junction.

PCV Post-capillary venule, through which lymphocytes enter the thymic veins and ultimately the blood.

HC Hassall's corpuscle; a structure peculiar to the thymus, in which epithelial cells become concentrically compressed and keratinized, possibly the site of removal of apoptotic cells. Although the function of Hassall's corpuscle remains unclear, it may have a role in the production of T^{REG} cells, regulatory cells that help to maintain tolerance to self (see Figs 15 and 22).

Selection Because of its importance and complexity, the process of selecting T lymphocytes for export has attracted intense study, and is currently considered to consist of the following stages.
1 CD4⁻CD8⁻ (double-negative) cells proliferate in the outer region of the cortex, during which they become CD4⁺CD8⁺ (double positive) and rearrange their TCR genes.
2 Under the influence of thymic stromal cells, T lymphocytes whose TCR recognizes one of the available 'self' MHC molecules (see Figs 11 and 12) survive, and the rest die.
3 Cells that recognize an MHC class I molecule lose CD4 and retain CD8; those that recognize an MHC class II molecule lose CD8 and retain CD4; thus they are now 'single positives'.
4 Under the influence of dendritic cells presenting 'self' antigens in the form of short peptides (for details see Fig. 18), potentially self-reactive T cells are eliminated.
5 The remainder, probably only about 2% of the starting population, are allowed to exit, and these make up the peripheral T-lymphocyte pool.

17 Secondary lymphoid organs and lymphocyte traffic

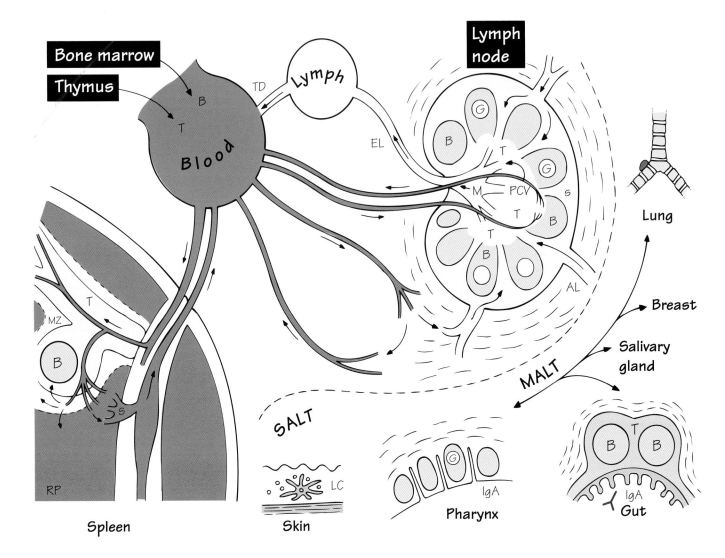

The ability to **recirculate** from blood to tissues and back through the lymphoid system is unique to lymphocytes and, coupled with their long lifespan and specificity for individual antigens, equips them for their central role in adaptive immune responses.

The thorough mixing of lymphocytes, particularly in the **spleen** and **lymph nodes**, ensures the maximum contact of antigen-presenting cells that have newly encountered antigen, with T and B lymphocytes potentially able to respond, which would otherwise be a very rare event. The body-wide dissemination of expanded T and B populations in readiness for a second encounter with the same antigen ensures that 'memory' is available at all sites.

Different types of lymphocyte 'home' to different regions in the lymphoid organs (**T** and **B** areas in the figure; B areas are shaded). This 'lymphocyte traffic' is regulated by a combination of chemotactic factors released from particular sites (mostly members of the chemokine family; see Fig. 7) and direct contact via adhesion receptors (sometimes known as 'addressins' because they direct

lymphocytes to particular sites in the body) between lymphocytes and the extracellular matrix or other cells such as the inner surface of the vascular endothelium or the dendritic antigen-presenting cells (not shown here, but see Fig. 8). The introduction of a new form of fluorescent microscopy, known as two-photon microscopy, has allowed the visualization of lymphocyte movement within living lymphoid tissue.

In general, lymph nodes respond to antigens introduced into the tissues they drain, and the spleen responds to antigens in the blood. The gut, lungs, breast and external mucous surfaces also have their own less specialized lymphoid areas that to some extent behave as a separate circuit for recirculation purposes and are often known as the **mucosa-associated lymphoid tissues** (MALT). These can be further subdivided into gut-associated (GALT), bronchial-associated (BALT) and skin-associated (SALT) lymphoid tissue. In each case, the objective seems to be to provide a local lymphoid system specialized for the antigens most likely to be encountered there.

Lymph node

Lymph nodes (or 'glands') constitute the main bulk of the organized lymphoid tissue. They are strategically placed so that lymph from most parts of the body drains through a series of nodes before reaching the thoracic duct (**TD**), which empties into the left subclavian vein to allow the lymphocytes to recirculate again via the blood.

AL, EL Afferent and efferent lymphatics, through which lymph passes from the tissues to first peripheral and then central lymph nodes. The cells found in afferent and efferent lymph are quite different. Naïve T cells enter lymph nodes from blood, but then leave via the efferent lymphatics, before eventually rejoining the blood. Memory or effector T cells enter tissues at sites of infection, and then travel back to lymph nodes via the afferent lymphatics. Afferent lymph also carries antigen and dendritic cells (known as veiled cells while in lymph) as they migrate from tissues such as the skin to the T-cell areas of the lymph node.

S Lymphatic sinus, through which lymph flows from the afferent lymphatic into the cortical and medullary sinuses. The lymph carries antigens and antigen-presenting cells from tissues to lymphoid tissue, and a series of fine collagen tubes runs from the cortical sinus into the T-cell areas, facilitating the movement of antigens directly to the antigen-presenting dendritic cells.

M Medullary sinus, collecting lymph for exit via the efferent lymphatic. It is in the medulla that antibody formation takes place and plasma cells are prominent.

G Germinal centre; an area of rapidly dividing cells that develops within the follicle after antigenic stimulation. It is the site of B memory-cell generation, and contains special follicular dendritic cells that retain antigens on their surface for weeks and perhaps even years (for further details see Fig. 19).

T T-cell area, or 'paracortex', largely occupied by T cells but through which B cells travel to reach the medulla. The dendritic cells here are specialized for presentation of antigen to T cells, and are probably the site where T and B lymphocytes of the right specificity meet and cooperate, which would otherwise be a very rare event.

PCV Post-capillary venule; a specialized small venule with high cuboidal endothelium (known as a high endothelial venule [HEV]) through which lymphocytes leave the blood to enter the paracortex and thence the efferent lymphatic, ultimately returning to blood via the thoracic duct.

Spleen

The spleen differs from a lymph node in having no lymphatic drainage, and also in containing large numbers of red cells. In some species it can act as an erythropoietic organ or a reservoir for blood.

T T-cell area; the lymphoid sheath surrounding the arteries is mostly composed of T lymphocytes.

B B-cell area, or lymphoid follicle, typically lying to one side of the lymphoid sheath. **Germinal centres** are commonly found in the follicle, alongside the follicular artery.

MZ Marginal zone; the region between the lymphoid areas and the red pulp, where lymphocytes chiefly leave the blood to enter the lymphoid areas, and red cells and plasma cells enter the red pulp.

RP Red pulp; a reticular meshwork through which blood passes to enter the venous sinusoids, and in which surveillance and removal of damaged red cells is thought to occur. For contrast, the lymphoid areas are sometimes called 'white pulp'. Macrophages in the red pulp and in the marginal zone can retain antigens, as the dendritic cells in the lymph nodes do. As in the medulla of the lymph node, plasma cells are frequent.

S Sinusoids; the large sacs that collect blood for return via the splenic vein.

Mucosa-associated lymphoid tissues

At least 50% of all tissue lymphocytes are associated with mucosal surfaces, emphasizing that these are the main sites of entry of foreign material. It is estimated that the total area of mucosal surfaces is 400 times that of the body, and that the number of bacteria colonizing these surfaces is many times more than the total number of cells in the body.

Gut The GALT is composed of two types of tissue: **organized** and **diffuse**. Typical organized tissues are the lymphoid aggregates, e.g. the Peyer's patches analogous to the lymphoid follicles in lymph nodes. The transfer of antigens from the gut lumen to the subepithelial area occurs via specialized M (membrane) cells, which pass them to dendritic cells where they are presented to T and B cells in the normal way. However, dendritic cells within the epithelium may also extend processes between the epithelial cells and take up antigens directly from the gut lumen. Although the ability to take up antigens is important in starting an adaptive immune response, some pathogens (e.g. HIV, *Salmonella*) may use this 'Trojan horse' route to invade their hosts.

Most of the B cells are specialized for IgA production, and B-cell memory develops in germinal centres. Cells that leave the follicles circulate in the blood to the diffuse lymphoid areas in the **lamina propria**, where large numbers of IgA plasma cells are found, as well as $CD8^+$ $\gamma\delta$ T cells, NK cells and mast cells. This preferential homing of MALT cells to MALT sites is mediated by specialized surface molecules on the lymphocytes and on the endothelium of blood vessel walls.

IgA Lamina propria B cells are responsible for the majority of IgA antibody, although a small amount is made in other sites such as bone marrow. IgA occurs mainly as dimers of two molecules held together by a J (joining) chain (see Fig. 14). IgA is protected against proteolytic digestion by a polypeptide **secretory piece** derived from the poly-Ig receptor and added to the IgA dimers in the epithelial cells.

Pharynx Lymphoid aggregates are prominent at this vulnerable site (tonsil and adenoids). The salivary glands also contain lymphocytes of MALT origin.

Lung The lung alveoli are largely protected from inhaled antigens by the upward movement of mucus propelled by beating cilia and ultimately coughed up or swallowed (the 'mucociliary escalator'). Organized and diffuse lymphoid tissues are present in the walls of the bronchi (the upper respiratory tract) but are absent from the lung alveoli (the lower respiratory tract). However, alveoli contain large numbers of alveolar macrophages that take up any debris or microorganisms that reach them. Alveolar macrophages can rapidly recruit T lymphocytes if an infection develops.

Skin Antigens entering via the skin can reach the local lymph node by being taken up in Langerhans' cells (**LC**) or dermal dendritic cells, which then can pass from the skin to the node, where they settle in the T-cell areas. Alternatively, soluble antigens can travel directly via the lymphatics to the draining lymph nodes. The skin also contains specialized populations of T cells that have a rather limited range of specificities and may act as an initial barrier to infection.

18 Antigen processing and presentation

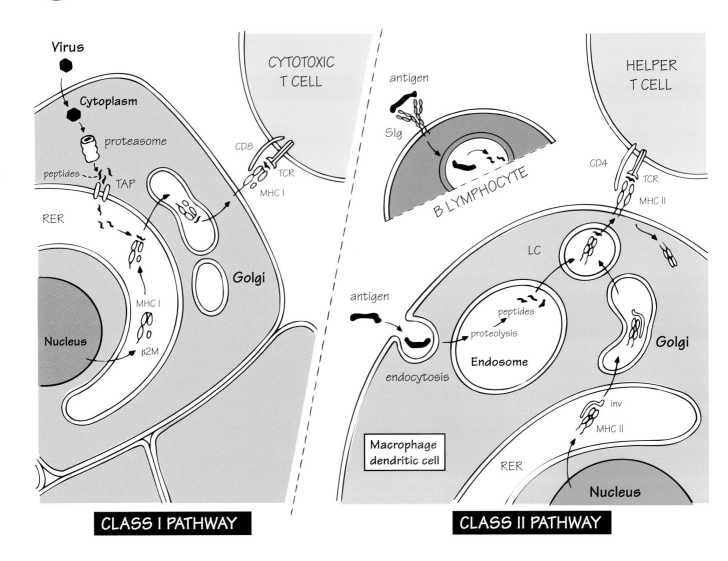

In discussing the MHC and the T-cell receptor (see Figs 11 and 12), frequent allusion has been made to the foreign peptides that bind to the former and are recognized by the latter. These peptides become associated with MHC molecules through two quite separate pathways (see figure), usually known for convenience as the class I pathway (left) and the class II pathway (right).

The first evidence that the MHC was involved in presenting antigens to T cells was the demonstration of 'MHC restriction' – the fact that T cells are specific for both antigen and MHC molecule. Then it was discovered that cytotoxic T cells could respond to viral nuclear antigens, which are not displayed on the surface of the virus! How could a T cell 'see' such a well-concealed antigen? The answer is shown in the left-hand figure above: virus-derived peptides become bound to class I MHC molecules inside the cell and are then transported to the surface, where T cells can recognize the peptide–MHC combination and, under appropriate circumstances, kill the virus-infected cell (for more details see Fig. 21).

At the same time, it was shown that a rather similar process occurs in the 'antigen-presenting' cells, mainly macrophages and dendritic cells, which activate helper T cells, with the difference that here it is the class II MHC molecules that transport the peptides to the surface (right-hand figure). This process is kept separate from the class I pathway by occurring in the endosomal/lysosomal vacuoles in which foreign material is normally digested (see Fig. 9). B lymphocytes can also process and present antigen, but only when they are able to bind it via their surface immunoglobulin (top right). Presentation by B cells to T cells is an essential step in **T-cell help** (see Fig. 19).

One can now appreciate that the real role of the MHC system is to transport samples of **intracellular proteins** to the cell surface for T cells to inspect them and react if necessary – by proliferating into clones and then helping macrophages or B cells or killing virus-infected cells, as described in the following pages.

The class I pathway

Virus Because they are synthesized in the cell, viral proteins are available in the cytoplasm, alongside self-proteins.

RER Rough endoplasmic reticulum, where proteins, including those of the MHC, are synthesized.

MHC I The single three-domain α chain associates with **β_2-microglobulin** to make a class I MHC molecule, whose structure is not fully stable until a peptide has been bound (see below). The efficient folding of MHC molecules around an antigen peptide requires a set of other 'chaperone' molecules found within the RER.

Proteasome A cylindrical complex of proteolytic enzymes with the property of digesting proteins into short peptides. This organelle has an essential role in regulating protein turnover in all cells. Its function has been hijacked by the immune system to provide peptides for class I MHC presentation. Two components of the proteasome that can alter its properties so as to produce peptides with better binding properties for MHC are encoded by the LMP genes that are found within the MHC region of the chromosome.

TAP TAP (transporter of antigen peptide) genes are found within the MHC region of the chromosome, and encode transporter proteins that carry the proteolytic fragments of antigen generated by the proteasome from the cytosol into the lumen of the endoplasmic reticulum where they bind to the peptide-binding groove of the class I MHC. Some viruses (e.g. human papillomavirus [HPV], Epstein – Barr virus [EBV], cytomegalovirus [CMV]; see Fig. 27) diminish immune recognition by encoding proteins that block TAP function or peptide binding to MHC.

Peptides of 8–10 amino acids are able to bind into the groove between the outer two α helices of the MHC molecule. If the peptides produced by the proteasome are too long special 'trimming' enzymes in the RER cut them to the right length. This binding is of high affinity but not as specific as that of antibody or the TCR. Thus, the six different types of class I MHC molecules on each cell (see Fig. 11) can between them bind a wide range of peptides, including many derived from 'self' proteins. Even after viral infection only a few percent of the available MHC molecules become loaded with viral peptides, and the rest will be derived from 'self' proteins from within the cell.

Golgi The Golgi complex, responsible for conveying proteins from the RER to other sites, including the cell surface.

TCR The T-cell receptor. Because of selection in the thymus (see Fig. 16), only a T cell whose receptor recognizes both the MHC molecule and the peptide bound in it will respond. This is a highly specific interaction, ensuring that cells displaying only 'self' peptides are not killed.

CD8 This molecule, expressed on cytotoxic T cells, recognizes the class I MHC molecule, a further requirement before killing of the virus-infected cell by the **cytotoxic T cell** can take place.

Cross-presentation Some antigens 'break the rules' and enter the class I processing pathway from the outside of the cell. Dendritic cells appear to be particularly efficient at cross presentation, which may be of importance in trying to stimulate an immunological response against tumours (see Fig. 42).

The class II pathway

Antigen Any foreign material taken in by phagocytosis or endocytosis will find itself in vesicles of the endocytic pathway, collectively known as **endosomes**, but including the acidic lysosomes, so that various digestive enzymes can act at the appropriate pH. In the case of microbial infection, the whole microbe is taken into the phagolysosome. Macrophages and dendritic cells carry many receptors on their surface (see Figs 3 and 5), which can bind sugars or other common constituents of pathogen surfaces and greatly increase the efficiency of uptake, by receptor-mediated uptake.

Sig Surface immunoglobulin allows the B lymphocyte to bind and subsequently endocytose antigen. Once within the cell, the antigen is processed in the usual way and peptides are presented on class II MHC. Because uptake is via a specific receptor, B cells selectively process only those antigens against which they carry specific antibody.

MHC II The two-chain MHC class II molecule forms a peptide-binding groove between the α1 and β1 domains, the β chain contributing most of the specificity. When first synthesized, this binding is prevented by a protein called the **invariant chain**, which is progressively cleaved off and replaced by newly produced peptides in the endosomes.

Inv (invariant chain) So called because, in contrast to the class II MHC molecules, it is not polymorphic. It acts as a 'chaperone' in helping MHC molecules to fold correctly as they are synthesized, and then binds to them, preventing peptides from associating with the peptide-binding site while still within the endoplasmic reticulum. It then directs the transport of the associated class II MHC molecules to specialized processing endosomes where, finally, it is proteolytically cleaved. This allows antigen peptides to bind the MHC, and allows the MHC carrying the peptides to exit the endosome and go to the cell membrane.

Peptides MHC class II molecules can bind peptides up to 20 amino acids long, which can extend out of each end. The peptides include some derived from microbes in the endosomes (e.g. persistent bacteria such as the tubercle bacillus), but also includes many self-peptides, some of which are derived from MHC molecules themselves. Peptides carrying post-translational modifications such as sugars or phosphate groups are also presented.

LC (class II loading compartment) Specialized acidic endosomes within which peptides are loaded on to the peptide-binding cleft of MHC class II molecules. The binding of peptides to MHC within this compartment is facilitated by two other class II-like molecules, HLA-DM and HLA-DO, which ensure that only those peptides with the best MHC fit are presented at the cell surface.

CD4 This molecule, expressed on **helper T cells**, interacts with MHC class II molecules, ensuring that the T-cell response (i.e. cytokine secretion; see Figs 21 and 23) is focused on an appropriate cell, i.e. either a B lymphocyte or a macrophage harbouring an intracellular infection. Thus, the type of T-cell response that occurs is determined by a sequence of factors: (i) the type of T cell (CD8 cytotoxic or CD4 helper); (ii) the class of MHC (I or II); (iii) the source of the peptide bound by the MHC (cytoplasmic or endocytosed); and, ultimately, (iv) the type of infection (viral or microbial). However, there are exceptions to this tidy scheme as described in Figs 26–32.

19 The antibody response

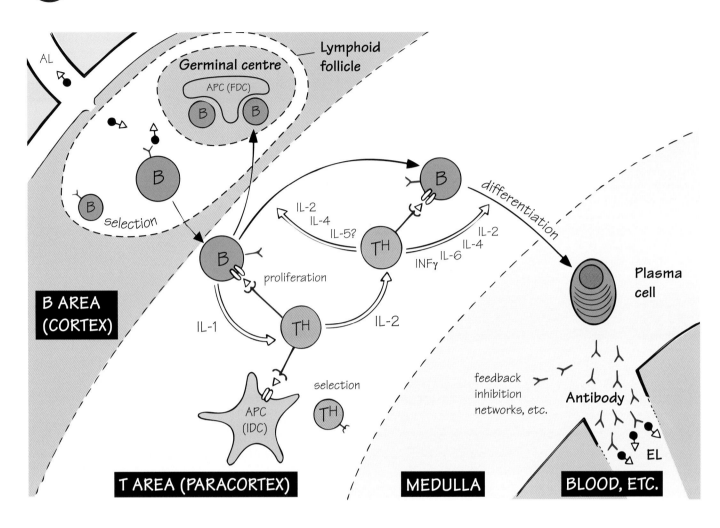

Animals born and reared in the complete absence of contact with any non-self material (not an easy procedure!) have virtually no immunoglobulins in their serum, but as soon as they encounter the normal environment, with its content of microorganisms, their serum immunoglobulin (Ig) rises towards the normal level of 10–20 mg (or about 60 000 000 000 000 000 molecules) per millilitre. This shows that immunoglobulins are produced only as a result of stimulation by foreign antigens, the process being known as the **antibody response**.

In the figure, these events are shown in a section through a stylized lymph node. Antigen is shown entering from the tissues (top left) and antibody being released into the blood (bottom right). The antigen is depicted as a combination of two components, representing the portion, or **determinant**, recognized by the B cell and against which antibody is eventually made (black circles) and other determinants that interact with T cells and are needed in order for the B cell to be fully triggered (white triangles). These are traditionally known as 'haptenic' and 'carrier' determinants, respectively. In practice, a virus, bacterium, etc. would carry numerous different haptenic and carrier determinants, whereas small molecules such as toxins may act as

haptens only. But even small, well-defined antigenic determinants usually stimulate a heterogeneous population of B cells, each producing antibody of slightly different specificity and affinity.

The main stages of the response are recognition and **processing** of the antigen (see Fig. 18), **selection** of the appropriate individual B and T cells (shown larger in the figure), **proliferation** of these cells to form a **clone**, and **differentiation** into the mature **functioning** state. A prominent feature of all stages is the many **interactions** between cells, which are mediated mostly by cytokines (white arrows in the figure). There are also a number of regulatory influences whose relative importance is not yet clear. Most of these cell interactions occur in the lymph nodes or spleen, but antibody can be formed wherever there is lymphoid tissue.

In a subsequent response to the same antigen, average affinity tends to be higher, precursor T and B cells more numerous and Ig class more varied. This **secondary** response is therefore more rapid and effective, and such an individual is described as showing **memory** to the antigen in question; this, for example, is the aim of most vaccines (see Fig. 41).

AL Afferent lymphatic, via which antigens and antigen-bearing cells enter the lymph node from the tissues (see Fig. 17).

APC Antigen-presenting cell. Before they can trigger lymphocytes, antigens normally require to be presented on the surface of a specialized cell. These cells form a dense network within lymphoid tissue, through which lymphocytes move around searching for antigen. B cells recognize antigen on the surface of follicular dendritic cells (FDC), while T cells interact with interdigitating dendritic cells (IDC) which carry high levels of MHC and **costimulatory** molecules.

FDC The follicular dendritic cell, specialized for presenting antigen to B lymphocytes in the B-cell follicles. Antigen on the surface of FDC is largely intact, maintaining its native conformation, and is often held in the form of antibody – antigen complexes that can persist for weeks or months.

IDC The interdigitating dendritic cell, specialized for presenting peptides to T cells in the T-cell area or paracortex. Some IDC develop directly within lymph node or spleen ('resident' dendritic cells) while others take up antigen in non-lymphoid tissues (those in skin epidermis, for example, are known as Langerhans' cells) by pinocytosis or phagocytosis, process it (see Fig. 18) and then migrate through the afferent lymphatics to the nearest lymph node.

Selection Only a small minority of lymphocytes will recognize and bind to a particular antigen. These lymphocytes are thus 'selected' by the antigen. The binding 'receptor' is surface Ig in the case of the B cell, and the TCR complex in the case of the T cell, which recognizes both antigen and MHC (see Figs 11 and 12).

Clonal proliferation Once selected, lymphocytes divide repeatedly to form a 'clone' of identical cells. The stimuli for B-cell proliferation are a variety of T-cell-derived cytokines and adhesion molecule interactions (see Fig. 12). T-cell proliferation is greatly augmented by another soluble factor (**IL-2**) made by T cells themselves. (For more information on interleukins see Figs 23 and 24.) The combination of selection by antigen followed by clonal proliferation has given to the whole lymphocyte response the descriptive name **clonal selection**. As the immune response progresses, B cells with higher and higher specificities are preferentially selected giving rise to **affinity maturation**.

Differentiation Once they have proliferated, B cells require help from T helper (T^H) cells to progress though further steps of differentiation. T-cell helper signals include both direct cell contact via receptors and their ligands (e.g. the interaction of CD40 on the T cell with CD40Ligand on the B cell) and soluble cytokines. An important aspect of differentiation is **isotype switching**, the ability of a B cell to produce a different class of antibody. Isotype switching is regulated mostly by specific interleukins. IgE production, for example, requires the release of IL-4 by a subset of T^H cells known as T^{H2} cells. Certain large repeating antigens can stimulate B cells without T-cell help; they are called 'T independent' and are usually bacterial polysaccharides. In the absence of T cell help (e.g. in certain genetic diseases in which CD40 or CD40L are absent) B cells secrete only IgM, and do not progress to isotype switching, memory cell formation or hypermutation.

Plasma cell In order to make and secrete antibody, endoplasmic reticulum and ribosomes are developed, giving the B cell its basophilic excen-

tric appearance. Plasma cells can release up to 2 000 antibody molecules per second. They stop circulating and are found predominantly in bone marrow or in the medulla region of lymphoid tissue. Most only live for a few days, but a much longer-lived subpopulation of plasma cells may also exist. Plasma cells can be chemically fused to tumor cells to form cellular hybrids. Some of these hybrids retain the tumour property of immortality, while continuing to produce their specific antibody. B-cell 'hybridomas' have been used to produce a huge array of monoclonal antibodies, which are now widely used in biology and medicine as molecular tools to isolate or classify molecules and cells. More recently, monoclonal antibodies are being used as drugs to treat cancer and autoimmunity, and potentially a range of other diseases.

EL Efferent lymphatic, via which antibody formed in the medulla reaches the lymph and eventually the blood for distribution to all parts of the body.

Memory cells Instead of differentiating into antibody-producing plasma cells, some B cells persist as memory cells, whose increased number and rapid response underlies the augmented secondary response, essentially a faster and larger version of the primary response, starting out from more of the appropriate B (and T^H) cells. Memory B cells differ slightly from their precursors (more surface Ig, more likely to recirculate in the blood) but retain the same specificity for antigen. The generation of memory B cells requires T cells, because T-independent responses do not usually show memory. T^H cells also develop into memory cells. Individual memory cells divide slowly (every few months) but do not appear to require antigen restimulation.

Germinal centres These are the major site of long-term antigen storage (primarily as complexes with antibody and complement, see Fig. 20) and of B-cell proliferation (**clonal expansion**). They are also the site for somatic hypermutation, a process that introduces small random mutations into the DNA sequence coding for the antibody binding site (see Fig. 13). While most of these mutations will decrease the specificity of the antibody for its antigen, some may increase it, and these will be selected for as the immune response continues, resulting in a general increase in antibody affinity (affinity maturation).

Feedback inhibition Antibody itself, particularly IgG, can inhibit its own formation, by binding the antigen and preventing it stimulating B cells. T cells that suppress antibody production have also been described (originally termed T^S, they are now more commonly called T^{REG}). Although these cells have still not been fully characterized (see Fig. 22), they act by regulating the T^H cell rather than by directly suppressing the B cell itself. In practice the single most important element in regulating antibody production is probably removal of the antigen itself.

Networks It was hypothesized by Jerne, and subsequently confirmed, that antibody idiotypes (i.e. the unique portions related to specificity) can themselves act as antigens, and promote both B-cell and T-cell responses against the cells carrying them, so that the immune response progressively damps itself out. This leads to the intriguing concept of a network of anti-idiotype receptors corresponding to all the antigens an animal can respond to – a sort of 'internal image' of its external environment. However, the actual role of networks in regulating ordinary antibody responses is not yet clear.

20 Antigen – antibody interaction and immune complexes

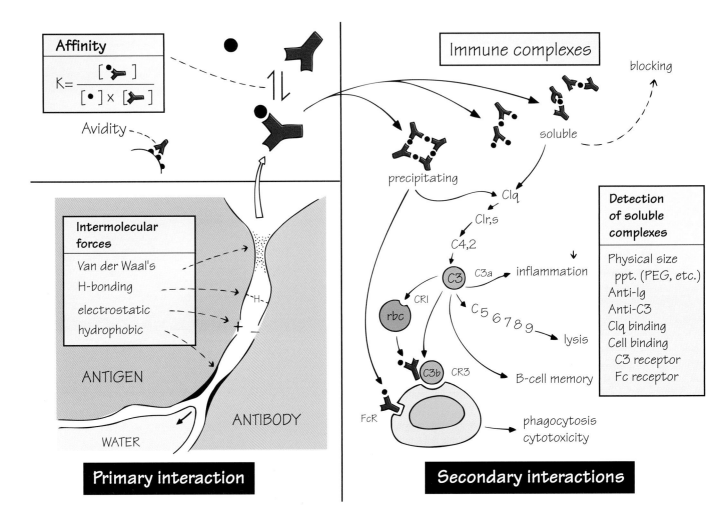

An antigen, by definition, stimulates the production of antibody, which in turn combines with the antigen. Both processes are based on **complementarity** (or 'fit') between two **shapes** – a small piece of the antigen (or **determinant**) and the **combining site** of the antibody, a cleft formed largely by the hypervariable regions of heavy and light chains (see Fig. 14). The closer the fit between this site and the antigenic determinant, the stronger the non-covalent forces (hydrophobic, electrostatic, etc., lower left) between them and the higher the **affinity** (top left). When both combining sites can interact with the same antigen (e.g. on a cell), the bond has a greatly increased strength, which in this case is referred to as 'avidity' (see Fig. 14).

The ability of a particular antibody to combine with one determinant rather than another is referred to as **specificity**. The antibody repertoire of an animal, stored in its V genes and expanded further by mutation (see Fig. 13), is expressed as the number of different shapes towards which a complementary specific antibody molecule can be made, and runs into millions.

What happens when antigen and antibody combine depends on the circumstances. Sometimes antibody alone is enough to neutralize the antigen. This is the case for toxins (such as tetanus or diphtheria) or microorganisms such as viruses that need to attach to cell-surface receptors in order to gain entry (the ability to block entry is often called neutralization).

Usually, however, a secondary interaction of the antibody molecule with another effector agent, such as complement or phagocytic cells, is required to dispose of the antigen. The importance of these secondary interactions is shown by the fact that deficiency of complement or myeloid cells can be almost as serious as deficiency of antibody itself (see Fig. 33).

The combination of antigen and antibody is called an **immune complex**; this may be small (soluble) or large (precipitating), depending on the nature and proportions of antigen and antibody (top right). The usual fate of complexes is to be removed by phagocytic cells, through the interaction of the Fc portion of the antibody with complement and with cell-surface receptors (bottom centre and see Figs 6 and 9). However, in some cases complexes may persist in circulation and cause inflammatory damage to organs (see Fig. 36) or inhibit useful immunity, e.g. to tumours or parasites.

Antigen – antibody interaction

The combining site of antibody is a cleft roughly $3 \times 1 \times 1$ nm (the size of five or six sugar units), although there is evidence that antigens may bind to larger, or even separate, parts of the variable region. Binding depends on a close three-dimensional fit, allowing weak intermolecular forces to overcome the normal repulsion between molecules. Although binding between antigen and antibody involves only non-covalent forces, and therefore is theoretically reversible, in practice the high **affinity** of most antibodies means that they rarely become detached from their targets before these are destroyed.

Van der Waal's forces attract all molecules through their electron clouds, but only act at extremely close range.

Hydrogen bonding (e.g. between NH_2 and OH groups) is another weak force.

Electrostatic attraction between parts of an antibody and antigen molecule with a net opposite charge (e.g. a negatively charged carboxyl group and a positively charged ammonium group) is sometimes quite strong.

Hydrophobic regions on antigen and antibody will tend to be attracted in an aqueous environment; this is probably the strongest force between them.

Affinity is normally expressed as the association constant under equilibrium conditions. A value of 10^5 L/mol would be considered low, while high-affinity antibody can reach 10^{10} L/mol and more, several orders of magnitude higher than most enzyme – substrate interactions. In practice, it is often **avidity** that is measured because antibodies have (at least) two valencies, and even with monovalent antigens a serum can only be assigned an average affinity. Average affinity tends to increase with time after antigenic stimulation, partly through cell selection by diminishing amounts of antigen, and partly via somatic mutation of Ig genes. High-affinity antibodies are more effective in most cases, but low-affinity antibodies persist too, and may have certain advantages (reusability, resistance to tolerance?).

Antigen It is remarkable that the process of making antibodies is so versatile that one can find antibodies specific for almost any type of molecular surface. These include the common components of pathogens such as proteins, nucleic acids, sugars and lipids, but also man-made synthetic molecules. For example, antibodies against amphetamines are being developed for the treatment of drug addiction.

Immune complexes

Under conditions of antigen or antibody excess, small ('soluble') complexes tend to predominate, but with roughly equivalent amounts of antigen and antibody, precipitates form, probably by lattice formation. Such precipitates activate the inflammatory response and probably underlie some types of occupational allergies, such as 'Farmer's lung' (see Figs 35 and 36). Complexes between antibodies and large antigens (e.g. nucleic acids) are associated with systemic autoimmune diseases such as systemic lupus erythematosus (SLE; see Fig. 38). In the presence of complement (i.e. in fresh serum) only small complexes are formed; in fact C3 can actually solubilize larger complexes (see also Fig. 36) and SLE is commonly associated with C2 and C4 deficiency.

Blocking of T-cell or antibody-mediated killing by complexes in (respectively) antigen or antibody excess may account for some of the unresponsiveness to tumours or parasite infections.

C1q the first component of complement, binds to the Fc portion of complexed antibody, possibly under the influence of a conformational change in the shape of the Ig molecule, although some workers hold that occupation of both combining sites (i.e. of IgG) is all that is needed. Activation of the 'classic' complement pathway follows.

Inflammation Breakdown products of C3 and C5, through interaction with mast cells, polymorphs, etc., are responsible for the vascular damage that is a feature of 'immune complex diseases' (see Fig. 36).

Lysis (e.g. of bacteria) requires the complete complement sequence. Sometimes the C567 unit moves away from the original site of antibody binding, activates C8 and 9, and causes lysis of innocent cells, (e.g. red cells); this is known as 'reactive lysis'.

Phagocytosis by macrophages, polymorphs, eosinophils, etc. is the normal fate of large complexes. In general, the antibody classes and subclasses that bind to Fc receptors also bind to complement, making them strongly opsonic, but the Fc and C3 receptors are quite distinct; IgM, for example, binds to complement much more than to cells. The majority of complexes in the circulation are picked up by red blood cells (**rbc** in figure) via their complement receptors (see Fig. 6). In transit through the liver and spleen, the complexes are removed by phagocytic cells.

Fc receptors (FcR) There are several types of receptor that bind the Fc constant part of antibodies. Some are found on phagocytes and facilitate uptake of IgG **opsonized** bacteria (see Fig. 9). Others are present on mast cells, and bind IgE. The interaction of IgE and specific antigen then triggers mast cell degranulation and allergic reactions (see Fig. 35). A different Fc receptor on B cells binds antibody – anigen complexes and acts to switch off further antibody production.

Cytotoxicity When antibody bound to a cell or microorganism makes contact with Fc receptors, the result may be killing rather than phagocytosis. Cells able to do this include macrophages, monocytes, neutrophils, eosinophils and natural killer cells (see Fig. 12).

B-cell memory Complement receptors on the follicular dendritic cells (see Fig. 19) help them to retain immune complexes and present the antigen to B cells in a way that, by selecting for mutants with high binding affinity, encourages the increase or 'maturation' of the affinity of the antibody response as a whole.

21 Cell-mediated immune responses

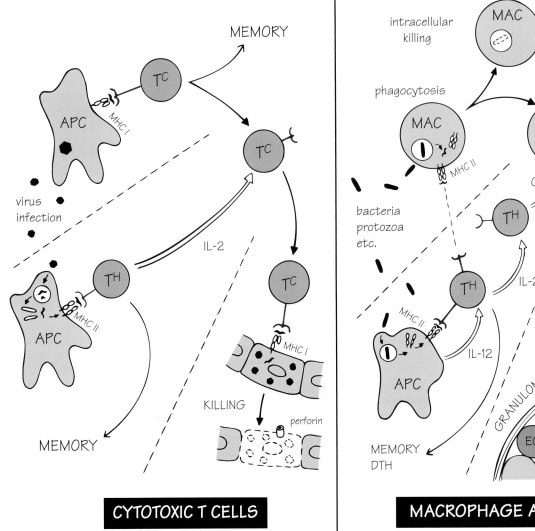

CYTOTOXIC T CELLS

MACROPHAGE ACTIVATION

Not all adaptive immunity involves antibody; protection against many important pathogens is mediated by T lymphocytes and B cells play no part. This type of immunity is often loosely termed 'cell-mediated immunity' (CMI) because, historically, it was not possible to transfer this immunity from one animal to another simply by transferring plasma containing antibodies. It was first identified in immunity to tuberculosis and later found to be also involved in contact sensitivity, immunity to some viruses, graft rejection, chronic inflammation and tumour immunity. CMI actually covers at least two different responses: the generation of specific **cytotoxic T cells** against intracellular viruses (left half of figure) and the effect of T cells in increasing the activities of 'non-specific' cells such as macrophages, to enable them to deal more vigorously with intracellular bacteria and other parasites (right half of figure). Confusingly, this latter type of response is often referred to as **delayed hypersensitivity**, which really only describes a particular kind of inflammatory tissue damage measured by skin testing. The role of CMI in causing tissue damage and the rejection of grafts is described in Figs 37 and 39, respectively.

Similar to the antibody response, CMI is regulated by various cells and factors (not shown in the figure), the normal function of which is presumably to limit damaging side effects, but which in some diseases seriously impair the protective response (see Fig. 22).

Viruses cannot survive for long outside the cells of the host, which they replicate in, spread from and sometimes destroy (see Fig. 27).

MHC I Class I MHC molecules (A, B, C in humans, K, D, L in mouse; see Fig. 11), which are an essential part of the recognition of viral antigens by the receptor on cytotoxic CD8 T cells (see Figs 12 and 18).

T^C The cytotoxic or 'killer' T cell with the function of detecting and destroying virus-infected cells. T^C release cytokines such as IFNγ and TNF-α, which may be important in controlling virus replication in cells without killing their targets. T^C are also important for controlling infections caused by some intracellular bacteria, especially *Mycobacterium tuberculosis*.

APC Although class I MHC is present on most cell types, thus allowing T^C to recognize and destroy any virally infected cells, T^C have first to be 'primed' by dendritic cells in the lymph nodes or spleen. Dendritic cells present viral antigens either by being infected directly, or by picking up fragments of neighbouring infected cells and loading them on to class I MHC (**cross-priming**).

T^H cells come in many types, and are required for almost all aspects of the immune response. For most antiviral responses, the T^C response is much more effective and long-lived if the virus also stimulates CD4 T^{H1} cells, which recognize viral antigens in association with class II MHC on the antigen-presenting cell. T^{H1} cells also have an important role in activating macrophages to become activated and kill intracellular pathogens (see T^{H1} and T^{H2} cells; see Fig. 15). A more recently described type of T^H cell, the T^{H17} cell, helps recruit and activate neutrophils. Individuals with defective T^{17} cells develop life-threatening fungal infections. Many of the functions of T^H are carried out by release of cytokines (especially IL-2 and IFNγ), which act at short range to activate their target cell (see below and Figs 23 and 24).

Killing Once primed and fully mature, T^C will specifically kill virally infected target cells. Killing occurs in two stages: **binding** by the receptor when it recognizes the right combination of class I MHC antigen plus virus, and Ca^{2+}-dependent **lysis** of the target cell. A key feature of all T-cell killing is that it works by activating the target cell to commit suicide, a process known as apoptosis (or programmed cell death). Once initiated, this process can continue after the T^C has detached, so that one T^C can kill several target cells. Killing is principally carried out by the secretion of **perforins** and **granzymes**. Perforins are small pore-forming molecules similar to the terminal complement lytic complex. Insertion of these molecules into the target cell membrane allows the entry of granzymes, proteolytic enzymes that activate the caspase cascade and thus initiate apoptosis. Some T^C use an alternative pathway, in which Fas ligand on the T cell (a molecule belonging to the TNF family) interacts with Fas receptor on the target, to initiate apoptosis.

Bacteria Certain bacteria, protozoa and fungi, having been **phagocytosed** by macrophages (MAC), avoid the normal fate of **intracellular killing** (see Fig. 9) and **survive**, either within the phagolysosome or free in the cytosol. In the absence of assistance from the T cells this would result in progressive and incurable infection. Note that the T-helper cells involved here need to secrete IFNγ and are therefore of the T^{H1} type. Recent research suggests that vitamin D is essential for IFNγ to activate macrophages effectively, perhaps explaining why

vitamin D deficiency has been associated with an increased risk of tuberculosis.

CK Cytokines, a large family of molecules produced by lymphoid and myeloid cells that regulate the activity of both haemopoietic and non-haemopoietic cells. Some of the main cytokines involved in cellular immunity are listed below (for more details see Figs 23 and 24).
• IL-1: an unusual cytokine in that it acts systemically through the body, activating the acute-phase response in liver (see Fig. 7) and increasing body temperature (fever) via its action on the hypothalamus.
• IL-2: once known as T-cell growth factor, IL-2 is important in allowing T cells to proliferate and differentiate into T^C. A structurally related cytokine, IL-15, promotes natural killer (NK) cell differentiation. Another member of the same family, IL-7, is essential for lymphocyte development (see Fig. 16).
• IL-12 and IL-23: two cytokines that share a common α chain; both are produced by dendritic cells and direct CD4 T cells towards the T^{H1} and T^{H17} differentiation pathway, respectively.
• IL-17: a more recently identified cytokine that is produced by the T^{H17} subset of T-helper cells. It stimulates a strong neutrophil response.
• MIF (macrophage migration inhibition factors): a heterogeneous group of molecules, which by restricting the movement of macrophages concentrate them in the vicinity of the T cell.
• MAF (macrophage activating factors): increase many macrophage functions, including intracellular killing and the secretion of various cytotoxic factors able to kill organisms **extracellularly**. The most important MAF is IFNγ.
• TNF-α: an important cytokine in the regulation of inflammation, via its effect on the properties of endothelium, causing leucocytes to adhere to the wall of the blood vessel and migrate into tissues. Like IL-1 it can act systemically, and if produced in excess can cause 'wasting', fever and joint destruction.
• IL-10 and TGF-β: in contrast to all the above, which enhance immune responses in various ways, these two cytokines are important in limiting and slowing down the cellular immune response, so as to avoid excessive damage to the infected tissues.

Granuloma Undegradable material (e.g. tubercle bacilli, streptococcal cell walls, talc) may be **sequestered** in a focus of concentric macrophages often containing some T cells, eosinophils (**EO**) and **giant cells**, made from the fusion of several macrophages. For the role of granulomas in chronic inflammation see Fig. 37.

Memory All the T cells involved in CMI can give rise to memory cells and thus secondary responses of increased effectiveness. Persistence of memory can apparently occur in the complete absence of antigen, although memory cells require cytokines such as IL-15 to continue dividing at a slow rate.

DTH Delayed-type hypersensitivity. The first evidence for adaptive immunity in tuberculosis was the demonstration (Koch, 1891) that injection of a tubercle antigen 'tuberculin' into the skin caused a swollen red reaction a day or more later. In patients with antibody, the corresponding reaction would take only hours, whence the terms 'delayed' and 'immediate' hypersensitivity, respectively. DTH depends on the presence of T-memory cells; the changes shown in the figure (right-hand side) occur at the site of injection, together with increased vascular permeability. Thus, DTH is a useful model of normal CMI and also a convenient test for T-cell memory.

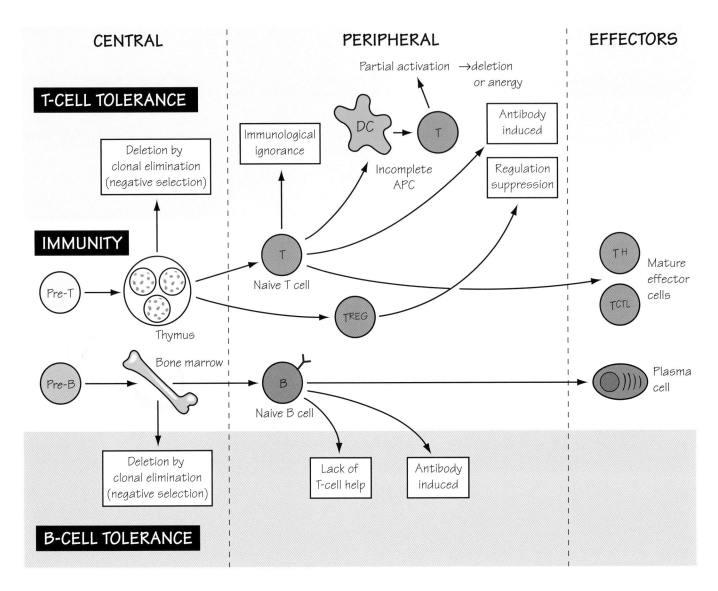

The evolution of recognition systems that initiate destruction of 'non-self' material obviously brings with it the need for safeguards to prevent damage to 'self'. This is a particularly acute problem for the adaptive immune system, because the production of T-cell and B-cell receptors involves an element of random gene rearrangement (see Figs 12 and 13), and therefore lymphocytes with receptors directed at 'self' will inevitably emerge in each individual. Furthermore, 'self' for one individual is not always the same as 'self' for another. For example, people of blood group A have red cells that carry antigen A but make antibodies to blood group B, and vice versa. The AB child of an A father and a B mother inherits the ability to make both anti-B and anti-A antibodies but must not make either, i.e. it must be **tolerant** to A and B.

Adaptive immunity, both B and T cell, in fact protects itself against possible self-reactivity at several stages (as shown in the figure). It used to be assumed that elimination of potentially self-reactive clones (negative selection) was the basis of all unresponsiveness to self, but many other regulatory mechanisms are now recognized. Nevertheless, self-tolerance is not absolute, and in some cases failure may lead to self-destructive immune responses (see Fig. 38).

In certain circumstances, normally antigenic 'non-self' materials can trigger these safeguarding mechanisms, a state known as **induced tolerance**, which might be very undesirable in some infections but very useful in the case of an organ transplant. The mechanisms involved in induced tolerance are likely to be very similar to those that maintain **self-tolerance**. Note that tolerance is by definition **antigen specific**, and quite distinct from the non-specific unresponsiveness induced by damage to the immune system as a whole, which is instead described as **immunodeficiency** (see Fig. 33).

Clonal elimination A cornerstone of Burnet's clonal selection theory (1959) was the prediction that lymphocytes were individually restricted in their recognition of antigen and that self-recognizing ones were eliminated early in life in the primary lymphoid organs. This is achieved for T cells by negative selection in the thymus (see Fig. 16), and for B cells in the bone marrow. Negative selection was first demonstrated convincingly for superantigens, such as those expressed by some mice endogenous retroviruses, because these delete a substantial proportion of T cells in the thymus. Neither B-cell nor T-cell deletion during development is complete, necessitating the existence of mechanisms of tolerance induction outside the primary lymphoid organs (**peripheral tolerance**).

Immunological ignorance Some antigens (e.g. those in the chamber of the eye) do not normally induce self-reactivity, simply because they never come into contact with cells of the normal immune system. This phenomenon is known as immunological ignorance. However, if the normal barriers are broken down, e.g. following injury or during a prolonged infection, these antigens can escape into the blood, and self-reactivity and damage of the tissue sometimes results.

Dendritic cells are thought to exist in both immature and mature states. Immature dendritic cells express MHC molecules but lack a full complement of costimulatory molecules such as CD80/86 or CD40 (see Fig. 18). Dendritic cells carry pattern recognition receptors (PRR; see Fig. 5), which recognize microbial products (such as the cell surface of bacteria) and trigger maturation. The processing and presentation of antigens, whether they be 'self' or 'non-self', by immature dendritic cells is thought to deliver a negative signal to T cells, and hence induce tolerance. In contrast, antigen presentation by mature dendritic cells results in full T-cell activation. The **danger hypothesis** postulates that both self-antigens and foreign antigens, administered in the absence of inflammation or pathogen-derived maturation stimuli, trigger tolerance. The hypothesis explains the old observation that **soluble antigen** is less immunogenic and more 'tolerogenic' than antigen administered in the presence of adjuvants, because it does not activate antigen-presenting cells to express the appropriate costimulatory molecules.

Negative signalling in T cells T cells express a number of molecules on their surface that transmit negative rather than activating signals. Engagement of these molecules (e.g. CTLA4, PD1) by ligands on the antigen-presenting cell surface serves to control and limit normal immune responses to prevent accidental collateral damage to self-tissues. However, this action may also limit the efficacy of an immune response, e.g. during chronic viral or bacterial infection or cancer. Antibodies to these molecules have shown promise for their ability to improve immune responses in these diseases, but the price may be the risk of some autoimmunity.

B-cell receptors (immunoglobulin) Exposure of B cells to high concentrations of antigen during their development leads to either clonal elimination (death of the B cell). B cells against self-antigens present at low concentrations (less than 10^{-5} mol/L) survive, but are never normally activated because they require help from T cells to trigger antibody secretion. This mechanism also guards against mature B cells that subsequently change their specificity because of somatic mutation of their V genes (see Figs 13 and 19) during an immune response. Thus, B-cell tolerance is determined by both 'central' tolerance (clonal deletion) and 'peripheral' tolerance (T-cell regulated).

T-cell receptors pass through an important selection process as they appear in the **thymus** (see Fig. 16), in which cells with receptors that have a sufficiently high affinity for self-peptides presented by thymic dendritic cells die by apoptosis and are therefore clonally deleted. Using transgenic technology, it is possible to create mice in which all B or T cells carry receptors of a single antigenic specificity. Despite the limitations of studying such artificial systems, these mice have been very important in clearly demonstrating clonal elimination and/or clonal anergy.

Regulatory T cells (T^{REG}, formerly known as suppressor T cells) T^{REG} cells that inhibit self-reactive lymphocytes are believed to differentiate during thymic development, and are characterized by the expression of CD4, CD25 (one chain of the IL-2 receptor) and a transcription factor, FoxP3. Elimination of these subpopulations of cells, either experimentally or genetically, leads to the development of widespread autoimmunity, emphasizing the importance of these cells in maintaining normal 'self' tolerance. Other types of T^{REG} can be induced, e.g. by administering antigens via the **oral** route, or by delivering repeated small doses of antigen. Regulatory or suppressive B cells have also been demonstrated. The mechanisms whereby regulatory cells inhibit their target (which is usually a T^H) can include the release of the inhibitory cytokines IL-10 and TGF-β, but other less understood mechanisms probably contribute. The balance between T^H and T^{REG} probably determines the eventual outcome of most immune responses and there is enormous interest in trying to expand populations of antigen-specific T^{REG} therapeutically so as to limit damaging autoimmune diseases (see Fig. 38).

Fetal (or neonatal) administration of antigen was the first method shown to induce tolerance. It probably operates by a combination of clonal elimination and deficient antigen presentation, due perhaps to antigen-presenting cell immaturity, although fetal B cells may also be particularly tolerizable because of differences in the way their Ig receptors are replaced (see above). There is some evidence that α-fetoprotein, a major serum protein in the fetus, can inhibit self-reactive T cells.

Oral route Antigens absorbed through the gut are first 'seen' by liver macrophages, which remove immunogenic aggregates, etc., leaving only soluble 'tolerogen'. In addition, antigen-presenting cells in the gut may be specialized for tolerance induction, to prevent immune responses against food. The gut epithelium contains large numbers of T^{REG} expressing suppressive cytokines such as IL-10 and TGF-β.

Antibody-induced tolerance Antibodies against some molecules on the surface of either T cells or antigen-presenting cells can help to induce a state of tolerance. Tolerance induced in this way is sometimes known as **enhancement**, from the ability to enhance the growth of tumours, transplants, etc. Antibodies to the CD4 molecule are particularly effective at inducing T-cell tolerance to antigens given at the same time.

High doses of antigen are usually more tolerogenic, although repeated low doses can also induce tolerance in T cells. As a rule, T-cell tolerance is easier to induce and lasts longer than B-cell tolerance.

Antigen suicide Antigens coupled to toxic drugs, radioisotopes, etc. may home in on specific B cells and kill them without exposing other cells to danger. A similar principle has been tried to eliminate tumour cells using toxins coupled to antibodies (see Fig. 42).

LIVERPOOL JOHN MOORES UNIVERSITY
LEARNING SERVICES

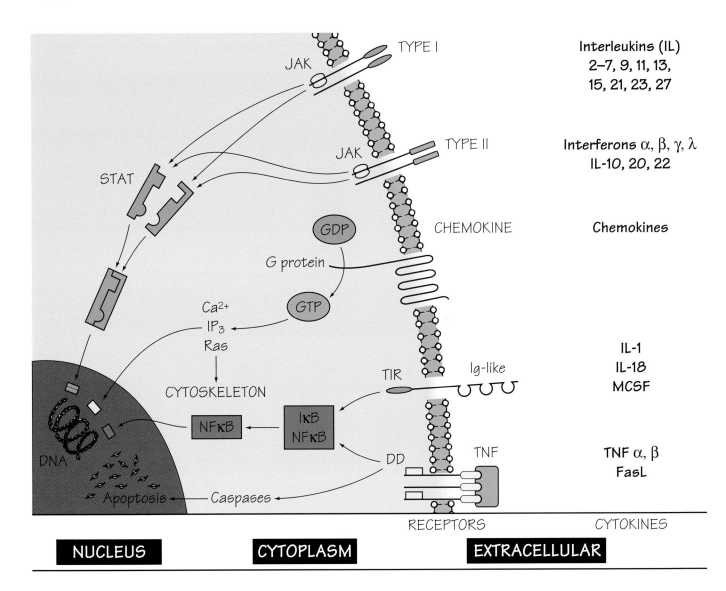

Virtually all immune responses involve cells communicating with each other – for instance T cells with B cells (see Figs 18 and 19) or T cells with macrophages (see Figs 18 and 21) – one cell sending signals to another to divide, differentiate, secrete antibody and so on. Cell–cell signalling can occur in two ways: the cells may come into contact, allowing receptor–receptor interactions (for some simple examples see Fig. 3) or a cell can secrete signalling molecules that travel to another cell, often in close proximity but sometimes at a distance.

Molecules that carry out this signalling function are known as **cytokines**. At least 30 of these are known, and the list can be extended if one includes every cell-derived molecule that acts on another cell. The term is usually restricted to molecules produced by cells with recognized immune function, such as lymphocytes, macrophages, dendritic cells, NK cells, even if some of them can also be made by, or act on, non-immunological cells. Cytokines are proteins of fairly low molecular weight (generally in the range MW 10000–80000) and they are completely distinct from that other major population of soluble immunological molecules, **antibody**, because they do not show any

specificity for antigen. Thus, predominantly the same cytokines would be involved in the immune response to measles, tuberculosis and malaria, unlike the situation with antibody.

For practical purposes, the main cytokines are classified into families (right), named after one of their functions, although sometimes the terminology is none too clear; e.g. one of the most important macrophage activators is called **gamma interferon** (IFNγ) because it, and the other interferons, were discovered through their effect in interfering with virus growth. In the same way **tumour necrosis factor** (TNF), despite its promising name, is chiefly involved in inflammation – and indeed can actually promote cancer. Most of the cytokines are now available in pure form, and are finding their way into medicine, although, as is the case with TNF, it can sometimes be more important to block their action.

Cytokine receptors are also classified into corresponding families, based on shared structure. These are shown in the figure (centre) with the intracellular pathways (left) by which cytokine–receptor binding leads to biological function. The following chapter describes some of these functions.

TNF Tumour necrosis factor, originally named for its ability in high doses to destroy some tumours but normally a major mediator of the inflammatory response (see Figs 7 and 24). TNF is made mainly by macrophages and most cell types carry receptors for it. The molecule is a trimer of three 17Mr polypeptides. Binding of TNF to its receptor can trigger either apoptosis or cell activation/survival via the NFκB pathway. TNF is the prototype of a family of about a dozen signalling molecules, some of which are secreted, while others (such as Fas) remain attached to the cell.

Interleukins A generic name often used interchangeably with cytokine.

IL-1 Although structurally different from TNF, interleukin 1 (IL-1) (and its homologue IL-18) also has a major role in inflammation. IL-1 is also responsible for fever, by acting on the temperature control centre in the hypothalamus. Its receptor belongs to the immunoglobulin superfamily (see Fig. 10) and shares an intracellular domain with the **toll receptors** of innate immunity (see Fig. 5). IL-1 production is regulated by the multimolecular complex called the **inflammasome** (see Fig. 5).

IL-2–IL-18 These molecules have a wide range of roles in innate and adaptive immunity (see table below and Fig. 24). Their two or three-chain receptors share cytokine-binding and/or signalling subunits, and are collectively known as type I receptors. Some interleukins (e.g. IL-3) have an important role in haemopoiesis, but confusingly some other molecules with related bone marrow activity are referred to as **colony-stimulating factors** (CSFs). These also bind to type I receptors, which are therefore sometimes known as **haemopoietin receptors**.

IFN Interferons IFNα and IFNβ are ubiquitous signals of innate immunity, which activate a broad range of antiviral mechanisms in many types of cell. They are produced by almost all cells, but plasmacytoid dendritic cells produce 1000 times more than any other cell type. In contrast, IFNγ is only weakly antiviral, but is a major regulator of macrophage activation. All three cytokines bind to type II receptors, and activate signals broadly similar to type I. The inhibitory cytokine IL-10 also binds to a type II receptor.

TGF-β Transforming growth factor β (not shown in figure). Named for its ability to induce non-adherent growth in cells in culture, TGF-β also inhibits the activity of T cells and macrophages and stimulates IgA production. Thus, like IL-10, it acts as an immunoregulatory molecule. TGF-β signals via members of the SMAD transcription factor family.

Chemokines A large family of molecules responsible for regulating cell traffic (see Fig. 7). Their receptors traverse the cell membrane seven times, a feature of receptors that act by coupling to GTP-binding (G) proteins. They are classified into two groups, CCR and CXC, depending on the spacing of two N-terminal cysteines, and are important (particularly CCR5) as coreceptors for HIV, the AIDS virus (see Fig. 28).

Apoptosis or programmed cell death is the process by which cells 'commit suicide'. It is important in organ development, the control of lymphocyte numbers, negative selection in the thymus, killing by NK and cytotoxic T cells. Induction of apoptosis by TNF involves activation of caspase enzymes, with eventual damage to mitochondria and degradation of DNA.

Fas, FasL Fas is a member of the TNF receptor family; Fas L is its ligand. Their binding triggers the process of apoptosis.

JAK, STAT Janus kinases (JAK) are receptor-associated kinases with two active sites (hence their name after the two-headed Roman god Janus). Binding of cytokines to type I or II receptors causes receptor dimerization, activation of the JAKs and subsequent recruitment and phosphorylation of signal transducers and activators of transcription (STATs). Activated STATs dimerize, migrate to the nucleus and switch on gene transcription. Molecular defects in the JAK–STAT pathway are associated with severe immunodeficiencies (see Fig. 33).

Ras Small GTP-binding proteins that regulate cytoskeleton, and hence cell shape and movement.

TIR Toll/interleukin receptor domain, common to toll-like receptors (see Fig. 5) and the IL-1 receptor and acting through the NFκB pathway to induce inflammation.

DD Death domains are signalling structures found within the intracellular section of TNF family of receptors. They are named for their part in activating apoptosis, but they also have a role in activating the NFκB pathway.

NFκB A transcription factor predominantly involved in inflammatory responses and also in counteracting apoptosis. It is normally held in check by an inhibitor, IκB (see Fig. 5).

The table below summarizes the main features of the best-studied cytokines.

Cytokine	Function	Cell of origin	Target
IL-1, IL-18	Inflammation, fever	Macrophage	Endothelium, hypothalamus, chondrocytes
IL-2, IL-15	Proliferation	T cells	T cells
IL-4, IL-13	IgE class switching	T^{H2} cells	B cells
IL-6	Inflammation, acute phase response, plasma cell formation	Macrophages	Liver, B cells
IL-8	Granulocyte infiltration	Multiple	granulocytes
IL-10	Suppression	T , B cells	Macrophages, dendritic cells, T cells
IL-12, IL-23	T^{H1} response	dendritic cells	T^{H1} cells
IL-17	T^{H17} response	T cells	granulocytes
TNF	Inflammation	Macrophage	Endothelium, macrophages
IFNα/β	Antiviral response	Plasmacytoid dendritic cells, multiple	All cells
IFNγ	T^{H1} response	T^{H1} cells	Macrophages
TGF-β	Suppression/tolerance	T^{REG} cells	T cells, macrophages

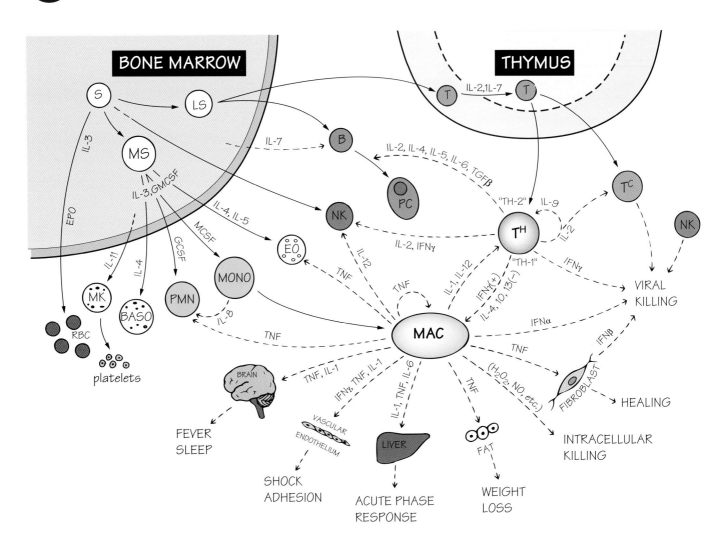

In the previous chapter cytokines were introduced as a collection of distinct molecules and receptors, but with a bewildering spectrum of regulatory effects on immunity and immune responses. Numerous cells can make one or several cytokines, depending on the circumstances. Very few cytokines are confined to a single function (pleiotropy) and very few functions rely on a single cytokine (redundancy). There are obvious advantages in this arrangement, for example the chance loss of a single cytokine or cytokine receptor gene would be unlikely to cause serious trouble – although there are exceptions to this (see Fig. 33). The analogy has even been made with language: one can communicate reasonably well with alphabets progessively lacking individual letters, but there would come a point where all messages would read the same. Many cytokines have related structures, and are thought to have evolved via repeated gene duplication (see Chapters 46 and 47). Presumably the present number of cytokines

and functions is what nature, through evolution, has found to be adequate without too much in the way of unwanted effects. Interestingly, some cytokines (e.g. interferons) are highly species-specific, others much less so.

The figure shows the combinations of cytokines responsible for the main pathways of immune cell development, differentiation, interaction and function, together with some of the side effects that can result from over-activity. As knowledge has accumulated, cautious attempts have been made to use cytokines in the clinic, although not many have yet become standard therapeutical agents. In fact, the most dramatic effects have come from blocking excessive cytokine activity, and both natural inhibitors and soluble receptors are being extensively tried out. At present, the amelioration of some cases of rheumatoid arthritis by anti-TNF antibodies is probably the best-known example; some others are mentioned on the opposite page.

Bone marrow (see also Figs 4 and 15). Unlike most other tissues of the body, the number of each type of immune cell varies greatly, depending on the amount of immune activity (hence the white blood cell count is often used as an indicator of disease; see Fig. 44). In addition, the turnover of cells in the immune system is very high (about 10^{10} neutrophils alone are formed and die each day in a healthy adult). Cytokines have a major role in regulating the proliferation, differentiation and commitment of immune and other blood cells from multipotent stem cells in the bone marrow. Some of these cytokines (stem cell factor, IL-7, IL-11) are made by bone marrow stromal cells, others (IL-3, IL-5, granulocyte macrophage colony-stimulating factor [GM-CSF], macrophage colony-stimulating factor [M-CSF], granulocyte colony-stimulating factor [G-CSF]) by T cells, macrophages or other tissues of the body. GCSF, which stimulates the development of granulocytes, is used to boost the production of neutrophils after bone marrow transplantation.

Immature **B lymphocytes** differentiate and proliferate in the bone marrow independently of antigen, in response to IL-7 and other cytokines. Once mature B cells have recognized their specific antigen, their differentiation into memory cells and plasma (antibody-producing) cells is controlled by cytokines from T helper (Th) cells such as IL-2, IL-4 and IL-6. Cytokines are particularly involved in Ig class switching, e.g. IL-4 for IgE, IL-5 and TGF-β for IgA.

Thymus Here T cells mature and are selected for MHC and antigen specificity (see also Figs 16 and 17). Thymic stromal cells produce cytokines of which IL-7 is the best known, but cell surface molecules known as *Notch* also play a part. The older concept of thymus **hormones** (e.g. thymosin) is still debatable.

T lymphocytes both secrete IL-2 and express receptors for it so that they can stimulate their own proliferation (autocrine); this molecule was formerly known as T-cell growth factor (TCGF). Different T-cell subsets go on to predominantly secrete different cytokines: Th1 cells activate macrophages via IFNγ, Th2 cells regulate B cells as described above, and the newly recognized Th17 subset activates polymorphonuclear leucocytes (PMN) via IL-17. Several T^{REG} subsets have been described, all with the ability to suppress Th cells. Interestingly, the expression of very high levels of one chain of the IL-2 receptor, CD25, is characteristic of regulatory T cells, and IL-2 deficiency leads preferentially to a deficit in regulatory T cells. The cytokines TGF-β and IL-10 mediate some of these activities. The differentiation of these different T subsets is itself regulated by cytokines: IL-12 secreted by dendritic cells, for example, favours T^{H1} development, IL-4 from mast cells favours T^{H2}, and IL-23 and TGF-β favour T^{H17} cells.

Macrophages act as key sentinels found within all organs of the body, releasing cytokines on contact with microbes which then initiate immune responses. Macrophages are the main source of the inflammatory cytokines TNF, IL-1 and IL-6. These cytokines are released into the blood stream, and act systemically, controlling the vasculature, the hypothalamus, muscle and liver. The antiviral cytokines IFNα and IFNβ are produced in very high amounts by a rare blood cell, the plasmacytoid dendritic cell.

Natural killer (NK) cells (see also Fig. 15). Their main function is to kill virus-infected and some tumour cells, but they are also important sources of IFNγ. Several cytokines are involved in their development (IL-12, IL-15) and activation (IL-12, IL-18, IFNα,β).

Microbial killing IFNα and β have a major role early in virus infections, both by damage to viral RNA and by enhancing MHC class I expression. Macrophage-derived TNF, IL-1 and IL-6 initiate the acute phase response, fever and, via IFNγ, the killing of intracellular microbes. In helminth infections Th2 cell-derived IL-4 and IL-5 are responsible for IgE production and eosinophilia, respectively.

Inflammation Here changes to vascular endothelium are critical, and TNF has a leading role, stimulating the increased production of adhesion molecules on the inner surface of blood vessels (see Fig. 7), the secretion of chemokines and the autocrine activation of macrophages. In severe infections or injuries, excessive TNF can get into the circulation, leading to shock and multiple organ damage. Type I acute inflammation (hypersensitivity) is interesting in that several relevant genes (IL-3, IL-4, IL-5, IL-9, IL-13) lie together on chromosome 5q (see Fig. 47), which is known to be a susceptibility locus for allergies.

Leucocyte migration Most leucocytes are very motile, not only circulating in blood, but leaving the blood, crossing the endothelium and migrating though lymphoid and non-lymphoid tissues. The chemokines have a key role in chemotaxis, the regulation of leucocyte traffic (e.g. attracting neutrophils, lymphocytes and monocytes to inflammatory sites) and the maintenance of the correct lymphoid architecture. The manipulation of chemokine pathways for therapy has so far been limited, partly because many of the chemokines have multiple and overlapping functions, and can bind to many different receptors.

Cytokines in therapy Early enthusiasm for cytokine treatment of tumours and infections, particularly HIV, has been dampened by severe side effects and, in many cases, ineffectiveness. At present the main cytokines in clinical use are IFNα for viral hepatitis, IFNα and IL-2 for certain tumours, notably renal, and IFNβ for treatment of multiple sclerosis. More dramatically successful is the use of cytokine antagonists (generally in the form of monoclonal antibodies) to control chronic inflammatory diseases, e.g. anti-TNF in rheumatoid arthritis. Anti-TNF is also under study for osteoarthritis, gout and heart failure. Disappointingly, it is only moderately beneficial in septic shock. An alternative approach is to use soluble receptors to block cytokine activity; the IL-1 receptor is the leading example.

25 Immunity, hormones and the brain

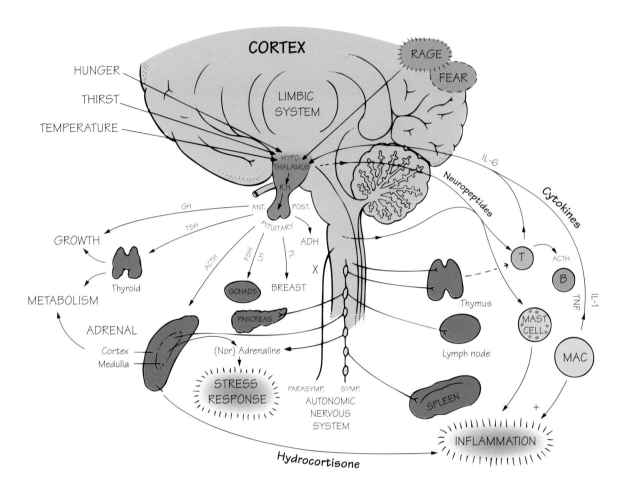

The language of immunology, with its emphasis on memory, tolerance, self and non-self, is reminiscent of that of neurology; indeed, the immune system has been referred to as a 'mobile brain'. Soluble 'messenger' molecules , the cytokines (see Figs 23 and 24), are used by immune cells to communicate with each other at short range across 'immunological synapses' closely parallelling the role of neutrotransmitters. Other long-range cytokines recall the hormone-based organization of the endocrine system, which is itself linked to the brain via the hypothalamic–pituitary–adrenal axis. Thus, it has been suggested that all three systems can be seen as part of a single integrated network, known as the psychoneuroimmunological, or neuroendocrinoimmunological, system.

Evidence to support this comes from several directions. Stress, bereavement, etc. are known to lower lymphocyte responsiveness, and the same can be achieved by hypnosis and, some claim, by Pavlovian conditioning. Lymphoid organs receive a nerve supply from both sympathetic and parasympathetic systems, and the embryonic thymus is partly formed from brain, with which it shares antigens such as theta. Lymphocytes secrete several molecules normally thought of as either hormones or neuropeptides (see bottom right of figure), while the effect of cytokines on the brain is well established (see Fig. 24).

The ability of the immune system to affect neurological and endocrine function is clearly established, and has a central role in several important diseases (see opposite page). The influence of the brain on immunological function remains more controversial and immunological opinion is divided as to its significance. At one extreme are those who dismiss the connections as weak, trivial and irrelevant. At the other are the prophets of a new era of 'whole body' immunology, stretching from the conscious mind to the antibody molecule, which would have significant implications for medical care. A middle-of-theroad view would be that such effects are the fine-tuning in a system that for the most part regulates itself autonomously. Time will tell who is nearest the truth.

 Immunology at a Glance, Tenth Edition. J.H.L. Playfair and B.M. Chain. © 2013 John Wiley & Sons, Ltd. Published 2013 by John Wiley & Sons, Ltd.

Central nervous system

Cortex The outer layer of the brain in which conscious sensations, language, thought and memory are controlled.

Limbic system An intermediate zone responsible for the more emotional aspects of behaviour.

Hypothalamus The innermost part of the limbic system, which regulates not only behaviour and mood but also vital physical functions such as food and water intake and temperature. It has connections to and from the cortex, brainstem and endocrine system.

Pituitary gland The 'conductor of the endocrine orchestra', a gland about the size of a pea, divided into anterior and posterior portions secreting different hormones (see below).

RH Specific releasing hormones produced in the hypothalamus stimulate the pituitary to release its own hormones, e.g. TRH (TSH-releasing hormone).

Neuropeptides Small molecules responsible for some of the transmission of signals in the CNS. The hypothalamus produces several that cause pain (e.g. substance P) or suppress it (e.g. endorphins, enkephalins).

Autonomic nervous system

In general, **sympathetic** nerves, via the secretion of noradrenaline (norepinephrine), excite functions involved in urgent action ('fight or flight') such as cardiac output, respiration, blood sugar, awareness, sweating. **Parasympathetic** nerves, many of which travel via cranial nerve **X** (the vagus), secrete acetylcholine and promote more peaceful activities such as digestion and close vision. Most viscera are regulated by one or the other or both. Massive sympathetic activation (including the adrenal medulla, see below) is triggered by fear, rage, etc. – the 'alarm' reaction, which if allowed to become chronic shades over into **stress**.

Endocrine system

Adrenal medulla The inner part of the adrenal gland, which when stimulated by sympathetic nerves releases **adrenaline** (epinephrine), with effects similar to noradrenaline but more prolonged.

Adrenal cortex The outer part of the adrenal gland, stimulated by corticotrophin (ACTH) from the anterior pituitary to secrete aldosterone, hydrocortisone (cortisol) and other hormones that regulate salt–water balance and protein and carbohydrate metabolism. In addition, hydrocortisone and its synthetic derivatives have powerful anti-inflammatory effects.

Thyroid Stimulated by thyrotrophin (TSH) from the anterior pituitary to release the iodine-containing thyroid hormones T_3 and T_4 (thyroxine), which regulate many aspects of cellular metabolism.

Growth hormone (GH) regulates the size of bones and soft tissues.

Gonads Two anterior pituitary hormones, follicle-stimulating hormone (FSH) and luteinizing hormone (LH), regulate the development of testes and ovaries, puberty and the release of sex hormones. These changes are especially subject to hypothalamic influence, e.g. psychological or, in animals, seasonal.

Breast Prolactin (PL) stimulates breast development and milk secretion.

Posterior pituitary Here the main product is antidiuretic hormone (ADH), which retains water via the kidneys in response to osmotic receptors in the hypothalamus.

The pancreas and parathyroids function more or less autonomously to regulate glucose and calcium levels, respectively, although the pancreas also responds to autonomic nervous signals.

Immune system

(*Note*: the elements shown in the figure are all considered in detail elsewhere in this book. Here, attention is drawn only to the features linking them to the nervous and endocrine systems.)

Cytokines The most convincing immune–nervous system link is the induction of fever by TNF, IL-1 and IFNs; high doses of many cytokines also cause drowsiness and general malaise. Cytokines, especially IL-2 and IL-6, are found in the brain. TNF and IL-1 are thought to induce ACTH secretion from the pituitary, probably via the hypothalamus.

Lymphoid organs Neurones terminating in the thymus and lymph nodes can be traced via sympathetic nerves to the spinal cord. Neuropeptides released within lymph nodes may regulate inflammation and dendritic cell function.

Lymphocytes have been shown to bear receptors for endorphins, enkephalins and substance P, and also to secrete endorphins and hormones such as ACTH. Small numbers of T lymphocytes are found naturally within the CNS and some studies suggest they may interact with macrophages to regulate both neuronal development and repair.

Immune responses are inhibited by hydrocortisone and sex hormones, and under stressful conditions, particularly when stress is inescapable, as with bereavement, examinations, etc. Hypnosis has been shown to inhibit immediate and delayed skin reactions. Whether corticosteroids can explain all such cases is a hotly debated point.

Autoimmunity It is remarkable how many autoimmune diseases (see Fig. 38) affect endocrine organs. Especially striking is the thyroid, where autoantibodies can both mimic and block the stimulating effect of TSH. Autoreactive T lymphocytes specific for myelin components have a key role in multiple sclerosis. The progress of this disease can be slowed by treatment with interferon β, and by Copaxone, an immunomodulatory drug that is thought to inhibit antigen presentation.

Immunity and psychological illness

A number of psychological illnesses have been linked to malfunction of immunity and/or vaccination, although it must be stressed that the links remain at best inconclusive.

Autism is a complex developmental disability of unknown cause that results in a range of behavioural and psychological symptoms. The condition usually manifests between the ages of 2 and 3, leading to the suggestion that the disease was caused by the MMR (measles, mumps and rubella) vaccine (see Fig. 41). Although the research leading to this suggestion has been completely discredited, and extensive epidemiological studies have failed to find any evidence to support any link between vaccination and autism, the publicity surrounding the research has caused a significant drop in the number of children vaccinated, leading to fears of a measles epidemic.

Myalgic encephalomyelitis/encephalopathy (sometimes known as chronic fatigue syndrome). A poorly defined condition characterized by extreme tiredness and exhaustion, problems with memory and concentration, and muscle pain. It may be associated with infection with unidentified viruses (it is sometimes referred to as postviral fatigue syndrome), because similar symptoms are often reported after infection with known viruses such as Epstein–Barr virus (EBV) (glandular fever) and influenza.

Gulf War syndrome A heterogeneous collection of psychological and physical symptoms experienced by soldiers involved in the Gulf War (1990–1), which some claimed was linked to the large number of vaccines given to recruits.

26 Antimicrobial immunity: a general scheme

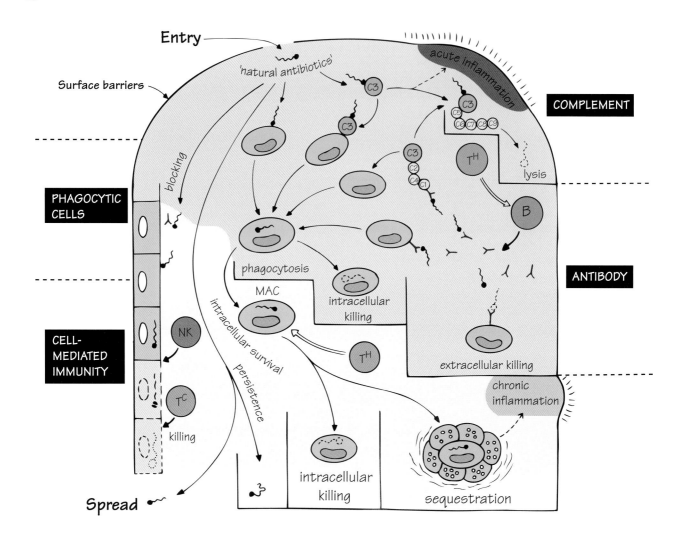

At this point the reader will appreciate that the immune system is highly efficient at recognizing **foreign** substances by their shape but has no infallible way of distinguishing whether they are **dangerous** ('pathogenic'). By and large, this approach works well to control infection, but it does have its unfortunate side, e.g. the violent immune response against foreign but harmless structures such as pollen grains, etc. (see Fig. 35).

Would-be parasitic microorganisms that penetrate the barriers of skin or mucous membranes (top) have to run the gauntlet of four main recognition systems: **complement** (top right), **phagocytic cells** (centre), **antibody** (right) and **cell-mediated immunity** (bottom), together with their often interacting effector mechanisms. Unless primed by previous contact with the appropriate antigen, antibody and cell-mediated (adaptive) responses do not come into action for several days, whereas complement and phagocytic cells (innate), being ever-

present, act within minutes. There are also (top centre) specialized **innate** elements, such as lysozyme, interferons, etc., which act more or less non-specifically, much as **antibiotics** do. Innate molecules that have evolved to block virus infection are sometimes called restriction factors.

Generally speaking, complement and antibody are most active against microorganisms free in the blood or tissues, while cell-mediated responses are most active against those that seek refuge in cells (left). But which mechanism, if any, is actually effective depends largely on the tactics of the microorganism itself. Successful parasites are those able to evade, resist or inhibit the relevant immune mechanisms, as illustrated in the following five figures. Evasion molecules, together with those that directly damage the host, are known as **virulence factors**. With increased knowledge of the host and pathogen genomes, identification of virulence factors has become a top priority.

Entry Many microorganisms enter the body through wounds or bites, but others live on the skin or mucous membranes of the intestine, respiratory tract, etc., and are thus technically outside the body.

Surface barriers Skin and mucous membranes are to some extent protected by acid pH, enzymes, mucus and other antimicrobial secretions, as well as IgA antibody (see below). The lungs, intestine, genitourinary tract and eye each have their own specialized combination of protection mechanisms.

Natural antibiotics The antibacterial enzyme **lysozyme** (produced largely by macrophages; see Fig. 29) and defensins, a family of polypeptides with broad antimicrobial properties, produced especially at mucosal surfaces, provide protection against many bacteria. Recent research has also discovered a whole range of molecules blocking viruses from becoming established in cells. These 'restriction factors' are regulated by the antiviral **interferons** (see Figs 24 and 27), soluble proteins released at sites of viral entry.

C3 Complement is activated directly ('alternative pathway') by many microorganisms, particularly bacteria, leading to their lysis or phagocytosis. The same effect can also be achieved when C3 is activated by antibody ('classic pathway'; see Fig. 6) or by mannose-binding protein.

T^H Helper T cells perform several distinct functions in the immune response to microbes. Some respond to 'carrier' determinants and stimulate antibody synthesis by B cells. Viruses, bacteria, protozoa and worms have all been shown to function as fairly strong carriers, although there are a few organisms to which the antibody response appears to be T-independent. Others secrete cytokines that attract and activate macrophages, eosinophils, etc. (see Figs 21 and 24), or enhance the activity of **cytotoxic T cells**. The central role of T helper cells in many infections is shown by the serious effects of their destruction, e.g. in AIDS (see Fig. 28).

B Antibody formation by B lymphocytes is an almost universal feature of infection, of great diagnostic as well as protective value. As a general rule, IgM antibodies come first, then IgG and the other classes; IgM is therefore often a sign of recent infection. At mucous surfaces, IgA is the most effective antibody (see Figs 14 and 17).

Blocking Where microorganisms or their toxins need to enter cells, antibody may block this by combining with their specific attachment site. Antibody able to do this effectively is termed 'neutralizing'. Vaccines against tetanus, diphtheria and polio all work via this mechanism, as does IgA in the intestine.

Phagocytosis by polymorphonuclear leucocytes or macrophages is the ultimate fate of the majority of unsuccessful pathogens. Both C3 and antibody improve this tremendously by attaching the microbe to the phagocytic cell through C3 or Fc receptors on the latter; this is known as 'opsonization' (see Fig. 9).

Intracellular killing Once inside the phagocytic cell, most organisms are killed and degraded by reactive oxygen species, lysosomal enzymes, etc. (see Fig. 8). In certain cases, 'activation' of macro

phages by T cells may be needed to trigger the killing process (see Fig. 21).

Extracellular killing Monocytes, polymorphs and other killer (K) cells can kill antibody-coated cells *in vitro*, without phagocytosis; however, it is not clear how much this actually happens *in vivo*.

NK Natural killer cells are able to kill many virus-infected cells rapidly, but without the specificity characteristic of lymphocytes. NK cells are activated by cells that lose expression of MHC class I molecules, a frequent characteristic of virus-infected cells and tumours that attempt to evade adaptive immune recognition in this way.

Intracellular survival Several important viruses, bacteria and protozoa can survive inside macrophages, where they resist killing. Other organisms survive within cells of muscle, liver, brain, etc. In such cases, antibody cannot attack them and cell-mediated responses are the only hope.

T^C Cytotoxic T cell, specialized for killing of cells harbouring virus, also allogeneic (e.g. grafted) cells (see Figs 21 and 39), and sometimes tumours (see Fig. 42).

Sequestration Microorganisms that cannot be killed (e.g. some mycobacteria) or products that cannot be degraded (e.g. streptococcal cell walls) can be walled off by the formation of a granuloma by macrophages and fibroblasts, aided by T^H-mediated immune responses (see Figs 21 and 37).

Spread Successful microorganisms must be able to leave the body and infect another one. Coughs and sneezes, faeces and insect bites are the most common modes of spread.

Persistence Some very successful parasites are able to escape all the above-mentioned immunological destruction mechanisms by sophisticated protective devices of their own. Needless to say, these constitute some of the most chronic and intractable infectious diseases. Major strategies for immune evasion include resistance to phagocytosis and/or intracellular killing, antigenic variation, immunosuppression and various forms of concealment.

Inflammation Although some microorganisms cause tissue damage directly (e.g. cytopathic viruses or the toxins of staphylococci), it is unfortunately true that much of the tissue damage resulting from infection is due to the response of the host. Acute and chronic inflammation are discussed in detail elsewhere (see Figs 7 and 37), but it is worth noting here that infectious organisms frequently place the host in a real dilemma: whether to eliminate the infection at all costs or to limit tissue damage and allow some of the organisms to survive. Given enough time, natural selection should arrive at the balance that is most favourable for both parasite and host survival.

Virulence factors include toxins, adhesion factors, resistance factors for antibiotics, enzymes that destroy immunological molecules, cytokine inhibitors, antigenic variation. Successful pathogens often possess many of these.

27 Immunity to viruses

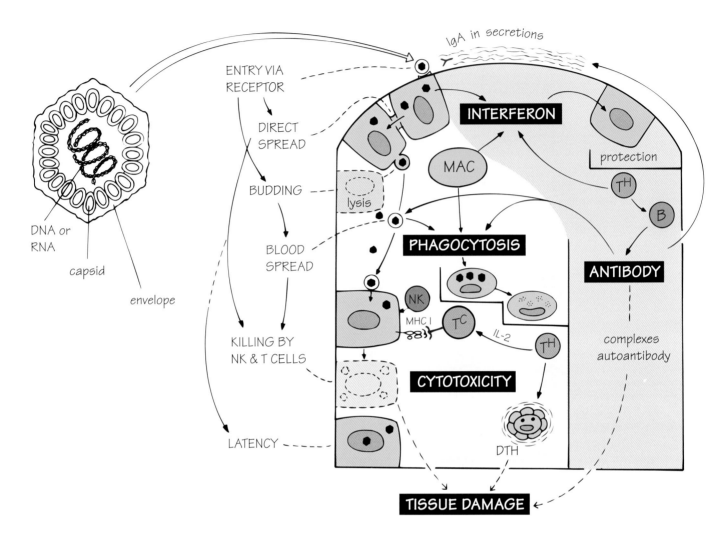

Viruses differ from all other infectious organisms in being much smaller (see Appendix I) and lacking cell walls and independent metabolic activity, so that they are unable to replicate outside the cells of their host. The key process in virus infection is therefore **intracellular replication**, which may or may not lead to cell death. In the figure, viruses are depicted as hexagons, but in fact their size and shape are extremely varied.

For rapid protection, **interferon** (top) activates a large number of innate mechanisms that can block viruses entering or replicating within cells. These molecules, collectively known as restriction factors, have the same 'natural antibiotic' role as lysozyme in bacterial infection, although the mechanisms are quite different. Antibody (right) is valuable in preventing entry and blood-borne spread of some viruses, but is often limited by the remarkable ability of viruses to alter their outer shape, and thus escape detection by existing antibody (the epidemics of influenza that occur each year are good examples of this mechanism at work). Other viruses escape immune surveillance by antibody by spreading from cell to cell (left). For these viruses the burden of adaptive immunity falls to the cytotoxic T-cell system, which specializes in recognizing MHC class I antigens carrying viral peptides from within the cell (see Fig. 18). However, many viruses (such as the herpes family) have evolved ways to escape cytotoxic T-cell recognition, by downregulating MHC expression, secreting 'decoy' molecules or inhibiting antigen processing. NK cells, which kill best when there is little or no MHC on the infected cell and come into action more rapidly than T^C cells, therefore have an important role.

Note that tissue damage may result from either the virus itself or the host immune response to it. In the long run, no parasite that seriously damages or kills its host can count on its own survival, so that adaptation, which can be very rapid in viruses, generally tends to be in the direction of decreased virulence. But infections that are well adapted to their normal animal host can occasionally be highly virulent to humans; rabies (dogs) and Marburg virus (monkeys) are examples of this ('zoonosis').

Intermediate between viruses and bacteria are those obligatory intracellular organisms that do possess cell walls (*Rickettsia*, *Chlamydia*) and others without walls but capable of extracellular replication (*Mycoplasma*). Immunologically, the former are closer to viruses, the latter to bacteria.

Receptors All viruses need to interact with specific receptors on the cell surface; examples include Epstein–Barr virus (EBV; CR2 on cells), rabies (acetylcholine receptor on neurones), measles (CD46 on cells) and HIV (CD4 and chemokine receptors on T cells and macrophages).

Interferon A group of proteins (see Figs 23 and 24) produced in response to virus infection, which stimulate cells to make proteins that block viral transcription, and thus protect them from infection.

T^C, NK, cytotoxicity As described in Figs 11, 18 and 21, cytotoxic T cells 'learn' to recognize class I MHC antigens, and then respond to these in association with virus antigens on the cell surface. It was during the study of antiviral immunity in mice that the central role of the MHC in T-cell responses was discovered. In contrast, NK cells destroy cells with low or absent MHC, a common consequence of viral infection.

Antibody Specific antibody can bind to virus and thus block its ability to bind to its specific receptor and hence infect cells. This is called neutralization and is an important part of protection against many viruses, including such common infections as influenza. Sometimes, viruses are able to enter cells still bound to antibody: within the cytoplasm, a molecule called TRIM21 binds antibody, and activates mechanisms that lead to rapid degradation of the virus–antibody complex.

Viruses

There is no proper taxonomy for viruses, which can be classified according to size, shape, the nature of their genome (DNA or RNA), how they spread (budding, cytolysis or directly; all are illustrated) and – of special interest here – whether they are eliminated or merely driven into hiding by the immune response. Brief details of a selection of important groups of viruses are given below.

Poxviruses (smallpox, vaccinia) Large; DNA; spread locally, avoiding antibody, as well as in blood leucocytes; express antigens on the infected cell, attracting CMI. The antigenic cross-reaction between these two viruses is the basis for the use of vaccinia to protect against smallpox (Jenner, 1798). Thanks to this vaccine, smallpox is the first disease ever to have been eliminated from the entire globe. However, stocks of vaccine against smallpox are once again being stockpiled in case this organism is spread deliberately as a form of bioterrorism.

Herpesviruses (herpes simplex, varicella, EBV, CMV [cytomegalovirus], KSHV [Kaposi sarcoma-associated herpes virus]) Medium; DNA; tend to persist and cause different symptoms when reactivated: thus, varicella (chickenpox) reappears as zoster (shingles); EBV (infectious mononucleosis) may initiate malignancy (Burkitt's lymphoma; see Fig. 42); CMV has become important as an opportunistic infection in immunosuppressed patients; and KSHV causes Kaposi's sarcoma in patients with AIDS (see Fig. 28). Some herpes viruses have apparently acquired host genes such as cytokines or Fc receptors during evolution, modifying them so as to interfere with proper immune function.

Adenoviruses (throat and eye infections) Medium; DNA. Numerous antigenically different types make immunity very inefficient and vaccination a problem. However, modified adenoviruses and adeno-associated viruses are being explored as possible gene therapy vectors, because they infect many cell types very efficiently.

Myxoviruses (influenza, mumps, measles) Large; RNA; spread by budding. Influenza is the classic example of attachment by specific receptor (neuraminic acid) and also of antigenic variation, which limits the usefulness of adaptive immunity. In fact the size of the yearly epidemics of influenza can be directly related to the extent by which each year's virus strain differs from its predecessor. Mumps, by spreading in the testis, can initiate autoimmune damage. Measles infects lymphocytes and antigen-presenting cells, causes non-specific suppression of CMI and can persist to cause SSPE (subacute sclerosing panencephalitis); some workers feel that multiple sclerosis may also be a disease of this type.

Rubella ('German measles') Medium; RNA. A mild disease feared for its ability to damage the fetus in the first 4 months of pregnancy. An attenuated vaccine gives good immunity.

Rabies Large; RNA. Spreads via nerves to the central nervous system, usually following an infected dog bite. Passive antibody combined with a vaccine can be life-saving.

Arboviruses (yellow fever, dengue) Arthropod-borne; small; RNA. Blood spread to the liver leads to jaundice.

Enteroviruses (polio) Small; RNA. Polio enters the body via the gut and then travels to the central nervous system where it causes paralysis and death. Within the blood it is susceptible to antibody neutralization, the basis for effective vaccines (see Fig. 41).

Rhinoviruses (common cold) Small; RNA. As with adenoviruses there are too many serotypes for antibody-mediated immunity to be effective across the whole population.

Hepatitis can be caused by at least six viruses, including A (infective; RNA), B (serum-transmitted; DNA) and C (previously known as 'non-A non-B'; RNA). In hepatitis B and C, immune complexes and autoantibodies are found, and virus persists in 'carriers', particularly in tropical countries and China, where it is strongly associated with cirrhosis and cancer of the liver. Treatment with IFNα or other antivirals can sometimes induce immunity and result in viral control. Very effective vaccines are now available for uninfected adults against hepatitis A and B.

Arenaviruses (Lassa fever) Medium; RNA. A haemorrhagic disease of rats, often fatal in humans. A somewhat similar zoonosis is Marburg disease of monkeys.

Retroviruses (tumours, immune deficiency) RNA. Contain reverse transcriptase, which allows insertion into the DNA of the infected cell. The human T-cell leukaemia viruses (HTLV) and the AIDS virus (HIV) belong to this group and are discussed separately (for details see Fig. 28).

Atypical organisms

Trachoma An organism of the psittacosis group (*Chlamydia*). The frightful scarring of the conjunctiva may be due to over-vigorous CMI.

Typhus and other *Rickettsia* may survive in macrophages, like the tubercle bacillus.

Prions These are host proteins which under certain circumstances can be induced to polymerize spontaneously to form particles called 'prions'. They are found predominantly in brain, and can cause progressive brain damage (hence their original classification as 'slow viruses'). The first example of a 'prion' disease was **kuru**, a fatal brain disease spread only by cannibalism. However, prion diseases are now thought to be responsible for scrapie and, most notoriously, for the UK epidemic of bovine spongiform encephalopathy (BSE or 'mad cow disease') and the human equivalent, Creutzfeldt–Jakob disease (CJD). Many aspects of prion disease remain poorly understood and there is no known treatment. There appears to be little or no immune response to prions, perhaps because they are 'self' molecules.

28 HIV and AIDS

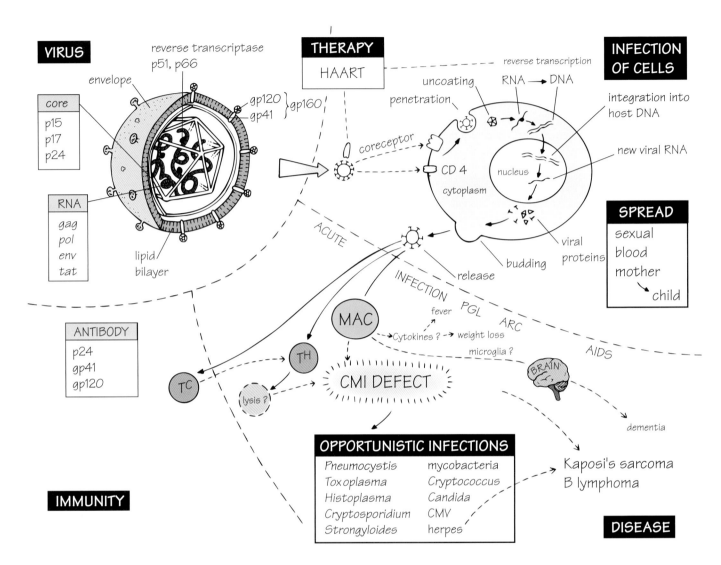

When in the summer of 1981 the Centers for Disease Control in the USA noticed an unusual demand for a drug used to treat *Pneumocystis* pneumonia, a rare infection except in severely immunosuppressed patients, and cases began to be increasingly reported in homosexual men, haemophiliacs receiving certain batches of blood products and drug users sharing needles, it became clear that a potentially terrible new epidemic had hit mankind, more insidious than the plague, more deadly than leprosy. The disease was baptized acquired immune deficiency syndrome (AIDS), and has become the most widely studied infectious disease of all time.

By 1984 the cause had been traced to a virus, now named HIV (human immunodeficiency virus), an RNA lentivirus (a subfamily of the retroviruses) that possesses the enzyme reverse transcriptase. This allows it to copy its RNA into DNA which is then integrated into the nucleus of the cells it infects, principally T-helper cells and macrophages. By processes still not fully understood, this leads to a slow disappearance of T-helper cells, with derangement of the whole immune system and the development of life-threatening opportunistic infections and tumours. The origin of HIV continues to be debated.

Attempts to link the epidemic to contaminated polio vaccine, or even to a political conspiracy have been totally discredited. The most likely hypothesis is that it spread from chimpanzees at some time during the twentieth century, perhaps due to human consumption of infected meat. Enormous effort has gone into trying to develop vaccines against HIV. HIV infection stimulates strong cellular immunity and antibody responses, but these responses never seem to be able to completely eliminate the virus, or even stop it dividing. In part, this may be because the virus infects T-helper cells, and hence blocks the development of full immunity. But the properties of HIV reverse transcriptase also give it an unusual ability to vary its antigens, which makes protective immunity or vaccination very difficult to attain.

HIV I and II, the AIDS viruses, closely related to the simian (monkey) virus SIV and more distantly to retroviruses such as HTLV I and II, which are rare causes of T-cell leukaemias. Their genome consists of double-stranded RNA. HIV II causes a much slower and less aggressive disease, and is predominantly found in Africa.

Immunology at a Glance, Tenth Edition. J.H.L. Playfair and B.M. Chain. © 2013 John Wiley & Sons, Ltd. Published 2013 by John Wiley & Sons, Ltd.

Gag The gene for the core proteins p17, p24 and p15. Like many viruses, HIV uses single genes to make long polyproteins which are then cut up by the virus's own enzyme (a protease) into a number of different functional units. Drugs that block this protease are an important class of HIV inhibitors.

Pol The gene for various enzymes, including the all-important reverse transcriptase.

Env The gene for the envelope protein gp160, which is cleaved during viral assembly to make gp120, the major structural protein of the viral envelope. Interaction with the **CD4** molecule found on T cells and macrophages, and a second interaction with a chemokine receptor (usually CCR5 or CXCR4), allows the virus to infect cells. About 1 in 10 000 Caucasian individuals have a homozygous deletion in CCR5, and these individuals are highly resistant to infection with HIV. *Gag, pol* and *env* genes are found in all lentiviruses.

Tat, rev, nef, vif, vpu Genes unique to HIV, which can either enhance or inhibit viral synthesis. Several of these molecules also antagonize cellular defence systems. For example, *nef* downregulates MHC class I and hence helps the virus escape immune detection, while *vif* blocks the enzyme APOBEC which destroys the viral RNA.

Reverse transcriptase is required to make a DNA copy of the viral RNA. This may then be integrated into the cell's own nuclear DNA, from which further copies of viral RNA can be made, leading to the assembly of complete virus particles which bud from the surface to infect other cells. A key feature of this enzyme is that it allows errors in transcription to occur (on average there is one base pair mutation for every round of viral replication). This feature allows the rapid evolution of new variants of virus during the course of an infection.

Acute infection A few weeks after HIV infection some patients develop a flu-like or glandular fever-like illness, although many remain symptomless. This is associated with a rapid rise in the level of virus in blood. During these weeks infected individuals rapidly develop antibody to HIV, which is routinely used for diagnosis. A very strong cellular T^C response also develops, which decreases the amount of virus in blood ('viral load') to a much lower, and sometimes undetectable, level. However, during this early phase there is also massive destruction of CD4 cells, predominantly in gut tissue. The mechanisms remain unclear.

Asymptomatic period Virus levels remain low for variable periods between a few months and more than 20 years. During this period infected individuals show few symptoms, although the number of $CD4^+$ T cells falls gradually. Despite this apparent 'latency', virus is in fact replicating rapidly and continuously, mainly within lymph nodes, and there is an enormous turnover of $CD4^+$ T cells, as infected cells die and are replaced. There may be a stage of progressive generalized lymphadenopathy (PGL).

Symptomatic period Patients develop a variety of symptoms, including recurrent *Candida* infections, night sweats, oral hairy leukoplakia and peripheral neuropathy (AIDS-related complex; ARC).

AIDS The full pattern includes the above plus severe life-threatening opportunistic infections and/or tumours. In some patients cerebral symptoms predominate. Almost every HIV-infected patient eventually progresses to AIDS. In 2009 there were estimated to be 33 million individuals infected with HIV worldwide, and over 2 million deaths from the disease, although the numbers of infected people appear to have reached a plateau. The vast majority of infected individuals are in sub-Saharan Africa, but there are expanding epidemics in many countries in the Far East. There are an estimated 1.5 million infected people in North America, 600 000–800 000 in western Europe and around 86 000 in the UK (many of them undiagnosed).

Kaposi's sarcoma A disseminated skin tumour thought to originate from the endothelium of lymphatics. It is caused by human herpes virus-8 (HHV-8, also known as KSHV), although it is still not clear why it is more common in AIDS than in other immunodeficient conditions.

T cells are the most strikingly affected cells, the numbers of $CD4^+$ (helper) T cells falling steadily as AIDS progresses, which leads to a failure of all types of T-dependent immunity. Although only 1% or less of T cells are actually infected, the virus preferentially targets memory cells.

MAC Macrophages and the related antigen-presenting cells, brain microglia, etc. are probably a main reservoir of HIV and are usually the initial cell type to become infected.

Transmission is still mainly by intercourse (heterosexual as well as homosexual), although in some areas infected blood from drug needles is more common. HIV can also be transmitted from mother to child at birth (vertical transmission) giving rise to neonatal AIDS. Not every exposure to HIV leads to infection, but as few as 10 virus particles are thought to be able to do so.

Pathology HIV is not a lytic virus, and calculations suggest that uninfected as well as infected T cells die. Many mechanisms have been proposed (including autoimmunity) but none is generally accepted.

Immunity The major antibody responses to HIV are against p24, p41 and gp120. Some antibody against gp120 is **neutralizing** but is very specific to the immunizing strain of virus. A strong CD8 T response against HIV-infected cells persists throughout the asymptomatic phase of HIV infection, suggesting that these cells are the major effector mechanism keeping HIV replication in check. Several innate mechanisms that may have a role in limiting lentivirus replication have been described (the molecules involved are often referred to as restriction factors). An RNA/DNA-modifying enzyme related to the one believed to be involved in somatic hypermutation (see Fig. 13) can provide protection by causing lethal mutations in viral nucleic acids. A cellular protein called TRIM5 acts at the stage of viral uncoating, while a membrane protein called tetherin inhibits the ability of newly formed virus to bud off from the cell surface. But HIV appears to have evolved ways of escaping all of them!

Therapy Early drugs used for treatment against HIV were inhibitors of viral reverse transcriptase, such as zidovudine (AZT). Treatment with a single drug provides only very short-term benefit as the virus mutates so fast that resistant strains soon emerge. However, the development of new families of drugs, e.g. against the HIV-specific protease, allowed the introduction of multidrug therapy, known as HAART (highly active antiretroviral therapy). Patients are treated with three, four or even more different antivirals simultaneously. These regimens have seen some spectacular successes in the clinic, leading to disappearance of AIDS-associated infections, and undetectable levels of virus for several years. However, this approach never results in permanent elimination of virus, and resistant strains eventually emerge. In any case the cost is prohibitive in most of the countries where HIV is common. Thus, the requirement for an effective HIV vaccine remains acute, and several trials aimed especially at stimulating a strong cellular response are under way.

29 Immunity to bacteria

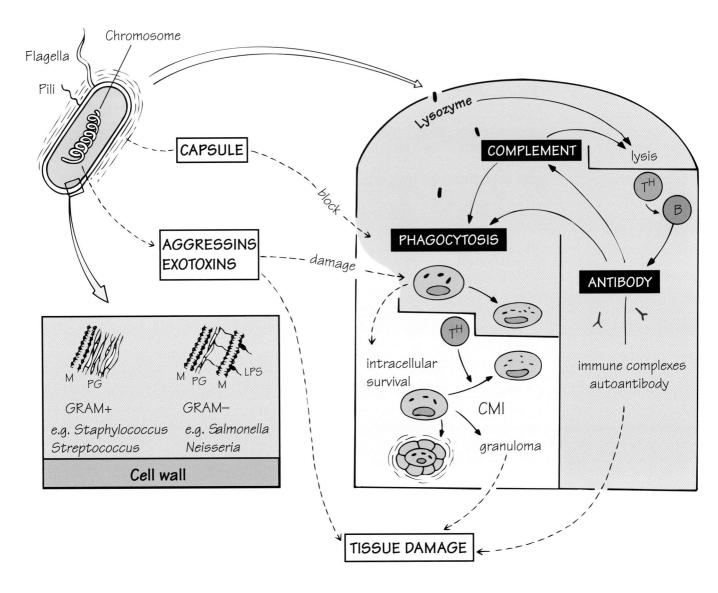

Unlike viruses, bacteria are cellular organisms, mostly capable of fully independent life, but some live on or in larger animals some or all of the time. Indeed, it is estimated that each human is colonized by some 10^{14} bacteria, equivalent to 10 bacteria for every cell of the body. This *microbiome* is made up of several thousand different species, most of which are innocuous and may even have a beneficial role in enhancing human health. However, a few species can cause disease and, together with viruses, these now constitute the major infectious threat to health in developed countries. Since the discovery of antibiotics, bacterial infection has been controlled largely by chemotherapy. However, with the recent rise in antibiotic-resistant strains of bacteria, there is renewed interest in developing new or improved vaccines against the bacteria responsible for such diseases as tuberculosis, meningitis and food poisoning.

The usual destiny of unsuccessful bacteria is death by **phagocytosis**; survival therefore entails avoidance of this fate. The main ways in which a bacterium (top left) can achieve this lie in the **capsule** (affecting attachment), the **cell wall** (affecting digestion) and the release of **exotoxins** (which damage phagocytic and other cells). Fortunately, most capsules and toxins are strongly antigenic and antibody overcomes many of their effects; this is the basis of the majority of antibacterial vaccines. In the figure, processes beneficial to the bacteria or harmful to the host are shown in broken lines. Bacteria living on body surfaces (e.g. teeth) can form colonies ('biofilms') which protect them against both immunity and antibiotics. As with viruses, some of the most virulent and obstinate bacterial infections are zoonoses – plague (rats) and brucellosis (cattle) being examples. Bacteria that manage to survive in macrophages (e.g. tuberculosis [TB]) can induce severe immune-mediated tissue damage (see Fig. 37).

Cell wall Outside their plasma membrane (M in the figure) bacteria have a cell wall composed of a mucopeptide called peptidoglycan (PG); it is here that **lysozyme** acts by attacking the *N*-acetylmuramic acid–*N*-acetylglucosamine links. In addition, Gram-negative bacteria have a second membrane with lipopolysaccharides (LPS, also called endotoxin) inserted in it. Bacterial cell walls are powerful inducers of inflammation, largely through their ability to activate the Toll-like receptors of innate immunity (see Figs 3 and 5).

Flagella, the main agent of bacterial motility, contain highly antigenic proteins (the 'H antigens' of typhoid, etc.), which give rise to immobilizing antibody. Some flagellar proteins activate the Toll-like receptor TLR5 (see Fig. 5).

Pili are used by bacteria to adhere to cells; antibody can prevent this (e.g. IgA against gonococcus).

Capsule Many bacteria owe their virulence to capsules, which protect them from contact with phagocytes. Most are large, branched, polysaccharide molecules, but some are protein. Many of these capsular polysaccharides, and also some proteins from flagella, are T-independent antigens (see Fig. 19). Examples of capsulated bacteria are pneumococcus, meningococcus and *Haemophilus* spp.

Exotoxins (as distinct from the **endotoxin** [LPS] of cell walls) Gram-positive bacteria often secrete proteins with destructive effects on phagocytes, local tissues, the CNS, etc.; frequently, these are the cause of death. In addition there are proteins collectively known as **aggressins** that help the bacteria to spread by dissolving host tissue.

Sepsis Occasionally, uncontrolled systemic responses to bacterial infection develop, which can lead to rapid life-threatening disease ('toxic shock'). Such responses are still an important cause of death after major surgery. Over-production of TNF-α, especially by macrophages, has a major role in these reactions.

Bacteria

Here, bacteria are given their popular rather than their proper taxonomic names. Some individual aspects of interest are listed below:

Strep *Streptococcus*, classified either by haemolytic exotoxins (α, β, γ) or cell wall antigens (groups A–Q). Group A β-haemolytic are the most pathogenic, possessing capsules (M protein) that attach to mucous membranes but that resist phagocytosis, numerous exotoxins (whence scarlet fever), indigestible cell walls causing severe cell-mediated reactions, antigens that cross-react with cardiac muscle (rheumatic fever) and a tendency to kidney-damaging immune complexes.

Staph *Staphylococcus*. Antiphagocytic factors include the fibrin-forming enzyme coagulase and protein A, which binds to the Fc portion of IgG, blocking opsonization. Numerous other toxins make staphylococci highly destructive, abscess-forming organisms. Large-scale use of antibiotics has caused the emergence of bacterial strains resistant to many antibiotics (methicillin-resistant *Staphyloccus aureus* [MRSA]), which are now proving a serious threat, particularly as hospital-acquired infections.

Pneumococcus (now S. pneumoniae), **meningococcus** Typed by the polysaccharides of their capsules, and especially virulent in the tropics, where vaccines made from capsular polysaccharides are proving highly effective in preventing epidemics. Also more common

in patients with deficient antibody responses (see Fig. 33). Chemical coupling of the capsular polysaccharides to a protein, such as diphtheria toxoid, converts these antigens from T-cell independent to T-cell dependent, thus greatly increasing memory and potency. Such conjugate vaccines have proven highly effective at preventing childhood meningitis and *Haemophilus* infection.

Gonococcus IgA may block attachment to mucous surfaces, but the bacteria secrete a protease that destroys the IgA; thus, the infection is seldom eliminated, leading to a 'carrier' state. Gonococci and meningococci are the only bacteria definitely shown to be disposed of by complement-mediated lysis.

Tuberculosis and leprosy bacilli These mycobacteria have very tough cell walls, rich in lipids, which resist intracellular killing; they can also inhibit phagosome–lysosome fusion. Chronic cell-mediated immunity results in the formation of granuloma, tissue destruction and scarring (see Fig. 37). In leprosy, a 'spectrum' between localization and dissemination corresponds to the predominance of cell-mediated immunity and of antibody, respectively. Tuberculosis is once again on the rise, partly as a result of increased travel, partly because of increased drug resistance and partly as a consequence of AIDS, and better vaccines to replace the only partially effective BCG (bacille Calmette–Guérin) are urgently being sought.

Escherichia coli is now perhaps the best-known bacterial species in the world, because of its ubiquitous use as a tool in all molecular biology laboratories. However, the species is a made up of an enormous number of different strains. Most are harmless inhabitants of the intestine of many mammals including humans, and may even be beneficial in supplying some vitamins and in suppressing the growth of other pathogenic bacteria. But a few strains produce exotoxins and have been responsible for major outbreaks of food poisoning. **Shigella** (causing dysentery) and **cholera** are two other examples of bacteria that grow only in the intestine, and are responsible for important human diseases.

Salmonella (e.g. *S. typhi*) also infects the intestine but can survive and spread to other parts of the body within macrophages. Recovery after infections may lead to a 'carrier' state.

Tetanus owes its severity to the rapid action of its exotoxin on the CNS. Antibody ('antitoxin') is highly effective at blocking toxin action, an example where neither complement nor phagocytic cells are needed.

Diphtheria also secretes powerful neurotoxins, but death can be due to local tissue damage in the larynx ('false membrane').

Syphilis is an example of bacteria surviving all forms of immune attack without sheltering inside cells. The commonly found autoantibody to mitochondrial cardiolipin is the basis of the diagnostic Wasserman reaction. Cross-reactions of this type, due presumably to bacterial attempts to mimic host antigens and thus escape the attentions of the immune system, are clearly a problem to the host, which has to choose between ignoring the infection and making autoantibodies (see Fig. 38) that may be damaging to its own tissues. **Borrelia**, another spirochaete, has the property (found also with some viruses and protozoa) of varying its surface antigens to confuse the host's antibody-forming system. As a result, waves of infection are seen ('relapsing fever'). **Brucella** may do the same.

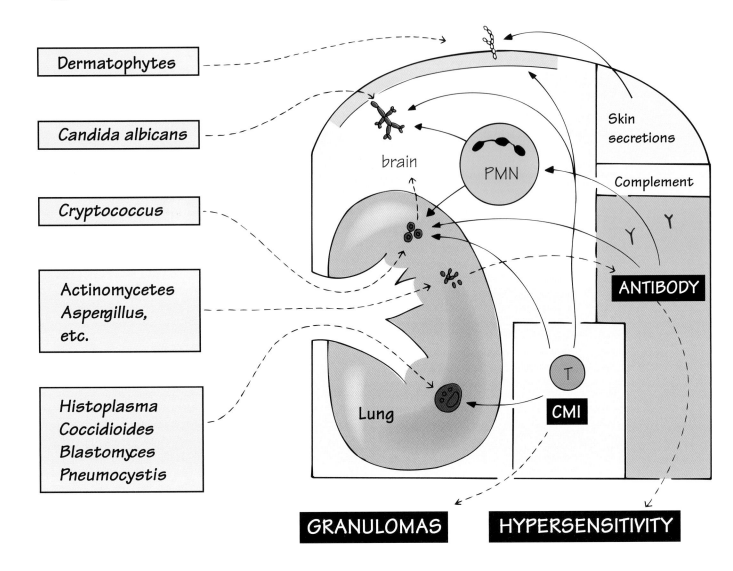

The vast majority of fungi are free-living, but a few can infect larger animals, colonizing the skin or entering via the lung in the form of spores (centre left). Fungal infections are normally only a superficial nuisance (e.g. ringworm, top), but a few fungi can cause serious systemic disease, particularly if exposure is intense (e.g. farmers) or the immune system is in some way compromised (e.g. AIDS); the outcome depends on the degree and type of immune response, and may range from an unnoticed respiratory episode to rapid fatal dissemination or a violent hypersensitivity reaction.

In general, the survival mechanisms of successful fungi are similar to those of bacteria: antiphagocytic capsules (e.g. *Cryptococcus*), resistance to digestion within macrophages (e.g. *Histoplasma*) and destruction of polymorphs (e.g. *Coccidioides*). Some yeasts activate complement via the alternative pathway, but it is not known if this has any effect on survival.

Perhaps the most interesting fungus from the immunological point of view is **Candida albicans** (upper left), a common and harmless inhabitant of skin and mucous membranes which readily takes advantage of any weakening of host resistance. This is most strikingly seen when polymorphs (PMN) or T cells are defective, but it also occurs in patients who are undernourished, immunosuppressed, iron deficient, alcoholic, diabetic, aged or simply 'run down' (see Fig. 33). Organisms that thrive only in the presence of immunodeficiency are called 'opportunists' and they include not only fungi, but also several viruses (e.g. CMV), bacteria (e.g. *Pseudomonas*), protozoa (e.g. *Toxoplasma*) and worms (e.g. *Strongyloides*), and their existence testifies to the unobtrusive efficiency of the normal immune system.

The most important ectoparasites ('outside living'; skin dwelling) are mites, ticks, lice and fleas. The last three are vectors for several major viral and bacterial diseases. The evidence for immunity, and the feasibility of a vaccine, are currently under intense study.

PMN Polymorphonuclear leucocyte ('neutrophil'), an important phagocytic cell. Recurrent fungal as well as bacterial infections may be due to defects in PMN numbers or function, which may in turn be genetic or drug-induced (steroids, antibiotics). Functional defects may affect chemotaxis ('lazy leucocyte'), phagolysosome formation (Chédiak–Higashi syndrome), peroxide production (chronic granulomatous disease), myeloperoxidase and other enzymes. Deficiencies in complement or antibody will of course also compromise phagocytosis (see also Fig. 33).

T As severe fungal infection in both the skin and mucous membranes (*Candida* spp.) and in the lung (*Pneumocystis* spp.) are common in T-cell deficiencies, T cells evidently have antifungal properties, but the precise mechanism is not clear. Some fungi (see below) can apparently also be destroyed by NK cells.

Hypersensitivity reactions are a feature of many fungal infections, especially those infecting the lung. They are mainly of type I or IV (for an explanation of what this means see Fig. 34).

Dermatophytes Filamentous fungi that metabolize keratin and therefore live off skin, hair and nails (ringworm). Sebaceous secretions help to control them, but CMI may also play an ill-defined part.

*Candida albicans (*formerly *Monilia)* A yeast-like fungus that causes severe spreading infections of the skin, mouth, etc. in patients with immunodeficiency, especially T-cell defects, but the precise role of T cells in controlling this infection is not understood. Dissemination may occur to the heart and eye.

Cryptococcus A capsulated yeast able to resist phagocytosis unless opsonized by antibody and/or complement (compare pneumococcus, etc.). In immunodeficient patients, spread to the brain and meninges is a serious complication. The organisms can be killed, at least *in vitro*, by NK cells.

Actinomycetes spp. and other sporing fungi from mouldy hay, etc. can reach the lung alveoli, stimulate antibody production and subsequently induce severe hypersensitivity ('farmer's lung'). Both IgG and IgE may be involved. *Aspergillus* sp. is particularly prone to cause trouble in patients with tuberculosis or cellular immunodeficiency. Dissemination may occur to almost any organ. The toxin (aflatoxin) is a risk factor for liver cancer.

Histoplasma (histoplasmosis), *Coccidioides* (coccidioidomycosis) and *Blastomyces* (blastomycosis) spp. are similar in causing pulmonary disease, particularly in America, which may either heal spontaneously, disseminate body-wide or progress to chronic granulomatosis and fibrosis, depending on the immunological status of the patient. The obvious resemblance to tuberculosis and leprosy emphasizes the point that it is microbial survival mechanisms (in this case, resistance to digestion in macrophages) rather than taxonomic relationships that determine the pattern of disease.

Pneumocystis jirovecii (formerly *P. carinii*) is mentioned here because although it was originally assumed to be a protozoan, studies of its RNA suggest that it is nearer to the fungi. *Pneumocystis* pneumonia has become one of the most feared complications of AIDS (see Fig. 28), which suggests that T cells normally prevent its proliferation, although the mechanism is so far unknown.

Ectoparasites

Mites are related to spiders. *Sarcoptes scabei* (scabies) burrows and lays eggs in the skin and induces antibody, but such protective immunity as there is appears to be cell-mediated (T^{H1}). The house dust mite *Dermatophagoides pteronyssinus* is an important cause of asthma. It induces high levels of IgE, and sublingual desensitization has had some success, probably by switching the T-cell response away from T^{H2} and towards the T^{H1} pattern. A DNA-based vaccine has been tried in mice.

Ticks, like mites, are arachnids, living on the skin and feeding on blood. They are vectors of several diseases, including Lyme disease, typhus and relapsing fever. A vaccine has had some success in cattle.

Lice (Pediculosis spp.) feed on skin, clinging to hairs. There are three main species, *P. capitis* (head lice), *Phthirius pubis* (pubic lice) and *P. corporis* (body lice). A vaccine has proved successful in salmon.

Fleas *Pulex irritans* is an important vector for plague, tularemia and brucellosis.

Mosquitoes and other vectors. Although not strictly parasites, mosquitoes should be mentioned as vectors for malaria, dengue, yellow fever and some forms of filariasis. Other important vectors are the sandfly (leishmaniasis), tsetse fly (trypanosomiasis), simulium fly (onchocerciasis) and reduviid bug (Chagas' disease).

31 Immunity to protozoa

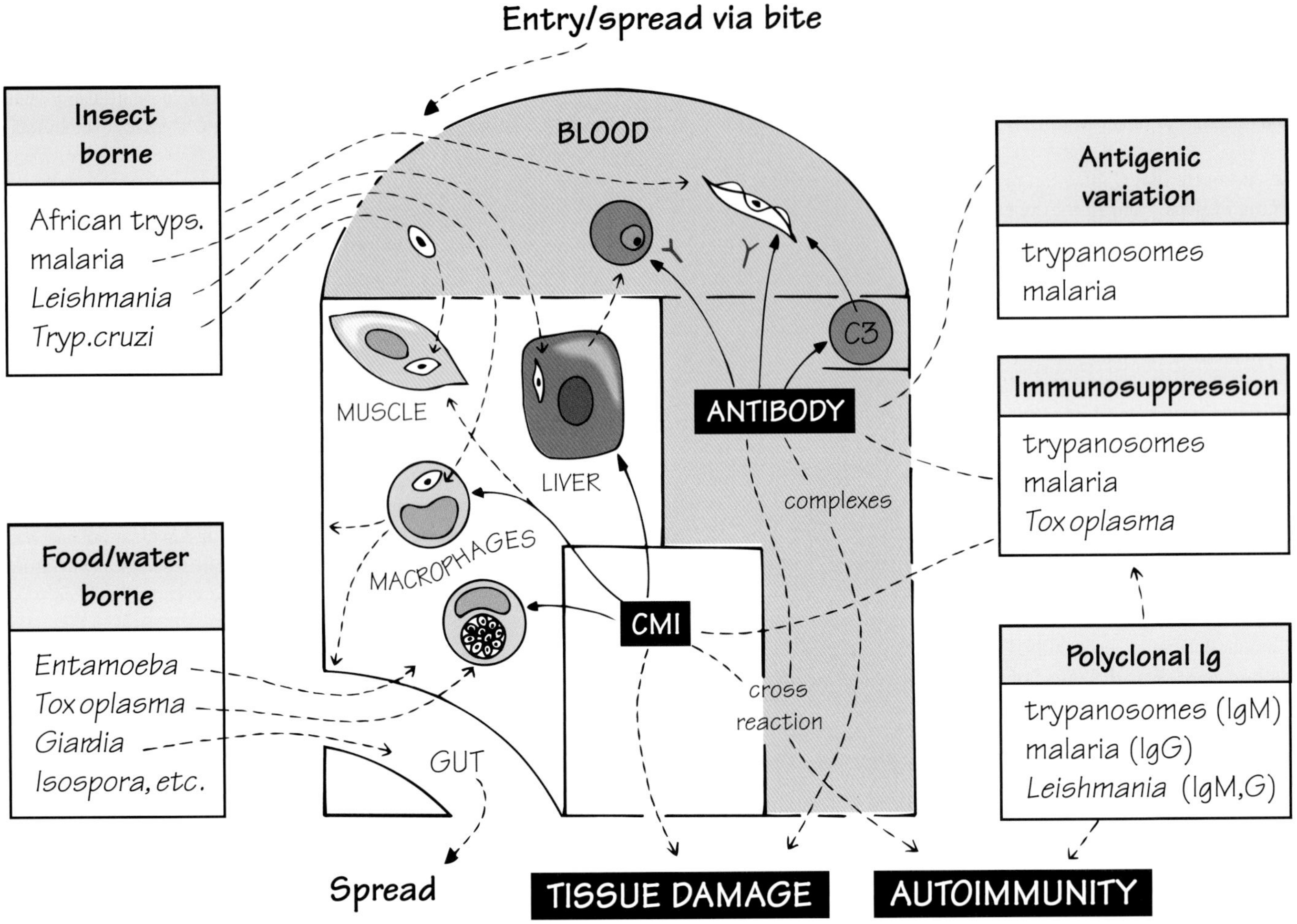

Relatively few (less than 20) species of protozoa infect humans, but among these are four of the most formidable parasites of all, in terms of numbers affected and severity of disease: malaria, the African and American trypanosomes, and *Leishmania* (top left). These owe their success to combinations of the strategies found among bacteria and viruses: long-distance **spread** by insect vectors (compare plague, typhus, yellow fever), **intracellular** habitat (compare tuberculosis, viruses), **antigenic variation** (compare influenza) and **immunosuppression** (compare HIV). However, these strategies are so highly developed that complete acquired resistance to protozoal infections is quite exceptional, and what immunity there is often serves merely to keep parasite numbers down ('premunition') and the host alive, to the advantage of the parasite. The rationale for vaccination is correspondingly weak, especially because some of the symptoms of these diseases appear to be brought about by the immune response rather than the parasite itself.

In contrast, the intestinal protozoa (bottom left) generally cause fairly mild disease, except when immunity is deficient or suppressed. Nevertheless, together with the intestinal worm infections described on the next page, they add up to a tremendous health burden on the inhabitants of tropical countries.

 Immunology at a Glance, Tenth Edition. J.H.L. Playfair and B.M. Chain. © 2013 John Wiley & Sons, Ltd. Published 2013 by John Wiley & Sons, Ltd.

African trypanosomes *Trypanosoma gambiense* and *T. rhodesiense*, carried by tsetse flies, cause sleeping sickness in West and East Africa, respectively. The blood form, although susceptible to antibody and complement, survives by repeatedly replacing its surface coat of glycoprotein 'variant antigen' by a gene-switching mechanism; the number of variants is unknown but large (perhaps as many as 1000). High levels of non-specific IgM, including autoantibodies, coexist with suppressed antibody responses to other antigens such as vaccines; this may be due to polyclonal activation of B cells by a parasite product (compare bacterial lipopolysaccharides). Humans are resistant to the trypanosomes of rodents because of a normal serum factor (high-density lipoprotein [HDL]) that agglutinates them – a striking example of innate immunity.

Malaria Malaria kills more than one million people each year, most of them children, and most of them in the world's poorest countries. *Plasmodium falciparum* (the most serious species), *P. malariae*, *P. vivax* and *P. ovale* are transmitted by female *Anopheles* mosquitoes. There is a brief liver stage, against which some immunity can be induced, probably via cytotoxic T cells, followed by a cyclical invasion of red cells, against which antibody is partially effective; antigenic variation, polymorphism and polyclonal IgG production may account for the slow development of immunity. Despite over 40 years of research, there is still no 100% effective vaccine (but see below). Vaccination protects against the red cell stage in certain animal models, and also against the sexual gamete state. Recently, a recombinant vaccine consisting of a sporozoite antigen fused to hepatits B surface antigen has shown real promise in African children. Human red cells lacking the Duffy blood group, or containing fetal haemoglobin (sickle cell disease), are 'naturally' resistant to *P. vivax* and *P. falciparum,* respectively. *P. malariae* is specially prone to induce immune complex deposition in the kidney. High levels of the cytokine TNF (see Fig. 24) are found in severe cases of malaria, and this may represent over-stimulation of macrophages by a parasite product – a form of pathology also seen in Gram-negative bacterial septicaemia (see Fig. 34). Malaria was one of the first diseases to be experimentally treated by the use of anti-TNF antibody, although without success so far; in fact TNF may also have a role in protective immunity.

Babesia **spp.,** or piroplasms, are tick-borne cattle parasites resembling malaria which occasionally infect humans, particularly following removal of the spleen or immunosuppressive therapy. In cattle and dogs an attenuated vaccine has been strikingly successful.

Theileria (East Coast fever), a cattle infection resembling malaria, except that the 'liver' stage occurs in lymphocytes, is unusual in being killed by cytotoxic T cells, i.e. it behaves essentially like a virus.

Leishmania A confusing variety of parasites, carried by sandflies, which cause an even more bewildering array of diseases in different parts of the tropics, although only in about 5% of exposed individuals. The organisms inhabit macrophages, and the pathology (mainly in the skin and viscera) seems to depend on the strength of cell-mediated immunity and/or its balance with antibody (compare leprosy). Cutaneous leishmaniasis in Africa is unusual in stimulating self-cure and subsequent resistance. This example of protection has apparently been known and applied in the Middle East for many centuries ('leishmanization'). There is evidence from mouse experiments that resistance is mediated by T^{H1} cells and can be compromised by T^{H2} cells, and also that nitric oxide (see Fig. 9) may be a major killing element.

Trypanosoma cruzi, the cause of Chagas' disease in Central and South America, is transmitted from animal reservoirs by reduviid bugs. It infects many cells, notably cardiac muscle and autonomic nervous ganglia. There is some suggestion that cell-mediated autoimmunity against normal cardiac muscle may be responsible for the chronic heart failure, and similarly with the nervous system, where uptake of parasite antigens by neurones and actual similarity between host and parasite have both been shown to occur. The organism has been killed *in vitro* by antibody and eosinophils, but the only prospect for vaccination seems to be against the blood stage. A better prospect would be to get rid of the poor housing in which the vector flourishes.

Toxoplasma **spp.** *T. gondii* is particularly virulent in the fetus and immunosuppressed patients, chiefly affecting the brain and eye. It can survive inside macrophages by preventing phagolysosome formation (compare tuberculosis), but cell-mediated immunity can overcome this. *Toxoplasma* stimulates macrophages and suppresses T cells, leading to varied effects on resistance to other infections.

Entamoeba histolytica normally causes disease in the colon (amoebic dysentery), but can move via the blood to the liver, etc., and cause dangerous abscesses by direct lysis of host cells. Some animals, and perhaps humans, may develop a degree of immunity to these tissue stages but not to the intestinal disease.

Giardia, Balantidium, Cryptosporidium, Isospora **spp.,** etc. normally restrict their effects to the gut, causing dysentery and occasionally malabsorption, but can be a severe complication of AIDS (see Fig. 28).

32 Immunity to worms

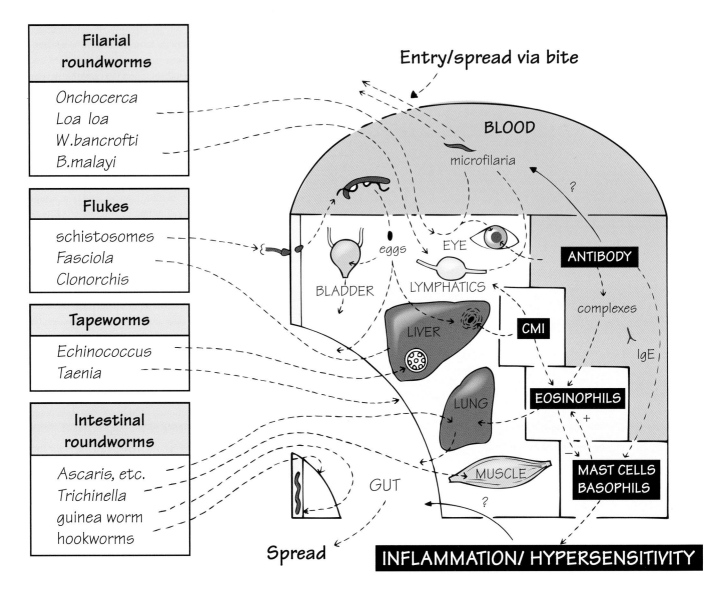

Parasitic worms of all three classes (roundworms, tapeworms and flukes) are responsible for numerous human diseases, including three of the most unpleasant (upper left): onchocerciasis, elephantiasis and schistosomiasis. These worms are transmitted with the aid of specific insect or snail vectors, and are restricted to the tropics, while the remainder (lower left) can be picked up anywhere by eating food contaminated with their eggs, larvae or cysts. A feature of many worm infections is their complex life cycles and circuitous migratory patterns, during which they often take up residence in a particular organ (see figure).

Another striking feature is the predominance of **eosinophils** and of **IgE**; as a result, hypersensitivity reactions in skin, lung, etc. are common, but whether they are ever protective is still controversial. As they do not replicate in the human host (unlike protozoa, bacteria and viruses), individual worms must resist the immune response particularly well in order to survive and, as with the best-adapted protozoa (compare malaria), immunity operates, if at all, to keep down the numbers of worms rather than to eliminate them. The outlook for vaccination might seem very dim, but it is surprisingly effective in certain dog and cattle infections.

Mystifying, but provocative, is the finding that several drugs originally used against worms (niridazole, levamisole, hetrazan) turn out to have suppressive or stimulatory effects on T cells, inflammation and other immunological elements, bringing out the point that worms are highly developed animals and share many structures and pathways with their hosts. Some very effective drugs against worms act against their nervous system.

Eosinophils may have three effects in worm infections: phagocytosis of the copious antigen–antibody complexes, modulation of hypersensitivity by inactivation of mediators and (*in vitro* at least) killing of certain worms with the aid of IgG antibody. Eosinophilia is partly due to mast-cell and T-cell chemotactic factors; T cells may also stimulate output from the bone marrow via cytokines such as IL-5.

IgE Worms, and even some worm extracts, stimulate specific and non-specific IgE production; it has been suggested but not proved that the resulting inflammatory response (e.g. in the gut) may hinder worm attachment or entry. There is also a belief that the high IgE levels, by blocking mast cells, can prevent allergy to pollen, etc. Production of IgE is considered to reflect the activity of T^{H2} helper cells.

Roundworms (nematodes)

Nematodes may be filarial (in which the first-stage larva, or microfilaria, can only develop in an insect, and only the third stage is infective to humans) or intestinal (in which full development can occur in the patient).

Filarial nematodes *Onchocerca volvulus* is spread by *Simulium* flies, which deposit larvae and collect microfilariae in the skin. Microfilariae also inhabit the eye, causing 'river blindness', which may be largely due to immune responses. In the Middle East, pathology is restricted to the skin; parasitologists and immunologists disagree as to whether this reflects different species or a disease spectrum (compare leprosy). *Loa loa* (loasis) is somewhat similar but less severe. *Wuchereria bancrofti* and *Brugia malayi* are spread by mosquitoes, which suck microfilariae from the blood. The larvae inhabit lymphatics, causing enormously enlaged limbs and/or scrotum (elephantiasis), partly by blockage and partly by inducing cell-mediated immune responses; soil elements (e.g. silicates) may also be involved. In some animal models, microfilaraemia can be controlled by antibody.

Intestinal nematodes (*Ascaris, Strongyloides, Toxocara* spp.). Travelling through the lung, larvae may cause asthma, etc., associated with eosinophilia. *Trichinella spiralis* larvae encyst in muscles. In some animal models, worms of this type stimulate good protective immunity. *Strongyloides* sp. has become an important cause of disease in immunosuppressed patients, suggesting that in normal individuals it is controlled immunologically. *Toxocara* sp., picked up from dogs or cats, is an important cause of widespread disease in young children, and eye damage in older ones.

Guinea worms (*Dracunculus*) live under the skin and can be up to 1.2 m long. **Hookworms** (*Ancylostoma, Necator* spp.) enter through the skin and live in the small intestine on blood, causing severe anaemia. None of these worms appear to stimulate useful immunity.

Flukes (trematodes)

Trematodes spend part of their life cycle in a snail, from which the cercariae infect humans either by penetrating the skin (*Schistosoma* sp.) or by being eaten (*Fasciola, Clonorchis* spp.). The latter ('liver flukes') inhabit the liver but do not induce protective immunity.

Schistosomes ('blood flukes') live and mate harmlessly in venous blood (*Schistosoma mansoni, S. japonicum*: mesenteric; *S. haematobium*: bladder), causing trouble only when their eggs are trapped in the liver or bladder, where strong granulomatous T-cell-mediated reactions lead to fibrosis in the liver and nodules and sometimes cancer in the bladder. The adult worms evade immune attack by covering their surface with antigens derived from host cells, at the same time stimulating antibody that may destroy subsequent infections at an early stage. Eosinophils, macrophages, IgG , IgE and the T^{H2} cytokines IL-4, IL-5 and IL-13, have all been implicated. Schistosomes also secrete a variety of molecules that destroy host antibodies and inhibit macrophages, etc., making the adult worm virtually indestructible. Nevertheless, there is evidence for the development of partial immunity, mainly directed at the skin and lung stages of the cycle. The combination of adult survival with killing of young forms is referred to as 'concomitant immunity'. An irradiated cercarial vaccine is effective in animals, but purified antigens are also being tried.

Fasciola spp. are chiefly a problem in farm animals, where they live in the bile duct. What immunity there is appears to lead mainly to liver damage and vaccines have been disappointing.

Clonorchis sp. infects humans but otherwise resembles *Fasciola* spp. It may lead to cancer of the bile duct.

Tapeworms (cestodes)

Cestodes may live harmlessly in the intestine (e.g. **Taenia spp.**), occasionally invading, and dying in, the brain ('cysticercosis'), or establish cystic colonies in the liver, etc. (e.g. the hydatid cysts of **Echinococcus spp.**), where the worms are shielded from the effects of antibody. Antigen from the latter, if released (e.g. at surgery) can cause severe immediate hypersensitivity reactions (see Fig. 35). An experimental vaccine has proved effective in dogs and sheep, the primary and intermediate hosts.

33 Immunodeficiency

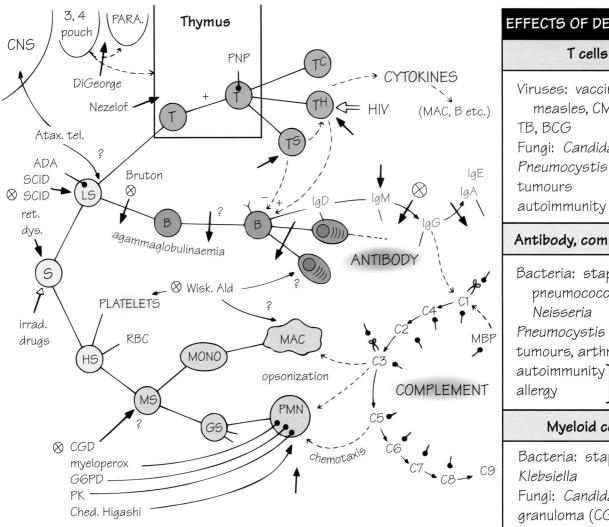

EFFECTS OF DEFICIENCY

T cells

Viruses: vaccinia
   measles, CMV
TB, BCG
Fungi: *Candida*
Pneumocystis
tumours
autoimmunity

Antibody, complement

Bacteria: staph., strep.
   pneumococcus
   Neisseria
Pneumocystis
tumours, arthritis
autoimmunity
allergy } (IgA)

Myeloid cells

Bacteria: staph., *E.coli*
Klebsiella
Fungi: *Candida*
granuloma (CGD)

Satisfactory immunity depends on the interaction of such an enormous variety of cells and molecules that inevitably a corresponding variety of different **defects** can reduce its efficiency, all with much the same end result: increased susceptibility to infection (right). There is a tendency for somewhat different patterns of disease according to whether the defect predominantly affects T cells (top), antibody and/or complement (centre) or myeloid cells (bottom).

Immunodeficiency may be **secondary** to other conditions (e.g. drugs, malnutrition or infection itself) or, less commonly, a result of **primary** genetic defects. It is remarkable how many of the latter are 'X-linked' (i.e. inherited by boys from their mothers; top left ⊗ in figure), suggesting that the unpaired part of the X chromosome carries several immunologically important genes (see Fig. 47). In some cases it appears that cell differentiation is interrupted at a particular stage (black arrows), but much more often there is a variable mixture of partial and apparently disconnected defects. The remarkable advances in genetics, and especially the ability to sequence enormous amounts of DNA, have resulted in a rapid increase in the number of diseases for which the missing gene product has now been identified (e.g. individual complement components, polymorph or lymphocyte enzymes (black circles), or cytokine receptor and adhesion molecules). Treatments being developed focus on replacement therapy, using either genes (gene therapy) or proteins. Although generally rare, these diseases have taught immunologists an enormous amount about the human immune system, providing 'experiments of nature' which complement and expand the many experimental genetic models developed in animals, especially rodents (for further details see Fig. 47).

The incidence of primary immunodeficiency depends on the definition of normality. Some scientists would argue that any manifestation of disease caused by infection reflects some level of immunodeficiency. Certainly both the frequency with which 'normal' people succumb to colds, sore throats and food poisoning etc. and the severity of the ensuing illnesses varies enormously between individuals. However, serious deficiency is found only in about one person per 1000.

Defects affecting several types of cell

Ret. dys. Reticular dysgenesis, a complete failure of stem cells, not compatible with survival for more than a few days after birth.

SCID Severe combined immunodeficiency, in which both T and B cells are defective. Some cases appear to be caused by deficiency of an enzyme, adenosine deaminase (**ADA**), which can be replaced by blood or marrow transfusion. Others result from a mutation in a cytokine receptor (the shared γ chain of the IL-2, IL-4 and IL-7 receptor). Recent gene therapy trials have used recombinant retroviruses to introduce the missing gene into bone marrow stem cells and have resulted in reconstitution of fully functional immune system. In a small number of children, however, tumours apparently caused by retroviral insertion have been reported. In some cases, HLA class I or II molecules are absent from lymphocytes ('bare lymphocyte syndrome').

Atax. tel. Ataxia telangiectasia, a combination of defects in brain, skin, T cells and immunoglobulin (especially IgA), apparently resulting from a deficiency of DNA repair.

Wisk. Ald Wiskott-Aldrich syndrome, a combination of eczema, platelet deficiency, and absent antibody response to polysaccharides. The genetic defect for this disease lies in a protein regulating cytoskeleton formation, but how this results in the pathology remains unclear.

Defects predominantly affecting T cells

DiGeorge syndrome: absence of thymus and parathyroids, with maldevelopment of other third and fourth pharyngeal pouch derivatives. Serious but very rare; it may respond to thymus grafting.

Nezelof syndrome: somewhat similar to DiGeorge syndrome but with normal parathyroids and sometimes B-cell defects.

PNP Purine nucleoside phosphorylase, a purine salvage enzyme found in T cells. Deficiency causes nucleosides, particularly deoxyguanosine, to accumulate and damage the T cell.

Cytokine defects, or defects in their receptors, appear to be rare, but IL-2 and IFNγ deficiency have been reported, as have individuals with deficiencies in the IL-12 receptor, and hence an inability to mount T^{H1} responses. Deficiencies in T^{H17} cells may lead to increased susceptibility to common and normally harmless fungal infections. There are also rare defects in several of the leucocyte adhesion molecules.

Defects predominantly affecting B cells

Agammaglobulinaemia or hypogammaglobulinaemia may reflect the absence of B cells (Bruton type), their failure to differentiate into plasma cells (variable types) or selective inability to make one class of immunoglobulin – most commonly IgA, but sometimes IgG or IgM. In X-linked hyper-IgM syndrome, there is a genetic defect in the CD40 ligand molecule on T-helper cells, which results in an inability to switch from making IgM to IgG.

Autoimmunity, allergies and polyarthritis are remarkably common in patients with antibody deficiencies, while both T- and B-cell defects appear to increase the risk of some tumours, especially those of the haemopoietic system.

Defects of complement

Virtually all the complement components may be genetically deficient; sometimes there is complete absence, sometimes a reduced level, suggesting a regulatory rather than a structural gene defect. In addition, deficiency of inactivators may cause trouble, e.g. C1 inhibitor (hereditary angio-oedema), C3b inhibitor (very low C3 levels). In general, defects of C1, C4 and C2 predispose to immune complex disease, particularly SLE, and of C5–9 to neisserial infection (meningococcal, gonococcal). C3 deficiency, as expected (see Fig. 6), is the most serious of all, and seldom compatible with survival. Low levels of mannose-binding protein (**MBP**) predispose to severe infections in children.

Defects affecting myeloid cells

CGD Chronic granulomatous disease, an X-linked defect of the oxygen breakdown pathway (see Fig. 9) usually involving a cytochrome, leads to chronic infection with bacteria that do not themselves produce peroxide (catalase positive) and with fungi such as *Aspergillus* spp. Gene therapy trials are in progress to try and replace the missing enzyme subunit. In a minority of cases there is another, non-X-linked, defect.

Myeloperoxidase, G6PD (glucose-6-phosphate dehydrogenase), **PK** (pyruvate kinase) and other polymorph enzymes may be genetically deficient, causing recurrent bacterial and fungal infection.

Ched. Higashi In the Chédiak–Higashi syndrome, the polymorphs contain large granules but do not form proper phagolysosomes. In other cases the response to chemotaxis is impaired ('lazy leucocyte').

Receptors of innate immunity

Genetic defects in several of these receptors (see Fig. 5) have now been reported, and more will undoubtedly be discovered. Some examples are **Toll-like receptor** 5 deficiency associated with susceptibility to Legionnaires' disease, **NOD-2** deficiency associated with Crohn's disease, and variations in the **mannose receptor** associated with susceptibility to leprosy and tuberculosis. Mutations in the interferon signalling pathway are associated with increased severity of common viral infections.

Secondary immunodeficiency

Age Immunity tends to be weaker in infancy and old age, the former being partly compensated by passively transferred maternal antibody. In the industrialized world, infection has become an important cause of illness and death in the elderly.

Malnutrition is associated with defects in antibody and, in severe cases, T cells; this may explain the more serious course of diseases (e.g. measles) in tropical countries. Both calorie and protein intake are important, as well as vitamins and minerals e.g. iron, copper and zinc.

Drugs can cause immunodeficiency, either intentionally (see Fig. 40) or unintentionally.

Infections Immunosuppression is found in a great variety of infections, being one of the major parasite 'escape' mechanisms (see Figs 27–32). **HIV** infection, by progressively destroying CD4 T cells, weakens the whole immune system (for more about AIDS see Fig. 28). Other viruses, such as measles, can temporarily depress T-cell function. Although this transitory effect may be of little consequence in the industrialized world, the increased susceptibility to common environmental pathogens, especially in food and water, is a major danger and cause of death to many children living in conditions of poor sanitation and hygiene in many other parts of the world. In all cases of T-cell deficiency, cell-mediated responses are of course reduced, but there are often secondary effects on antibody as well.

Tumours are often associated with immunodeficiency, notably Hodgkin's disease, myeloma and leukaemias; it is sometimes hard to be sure which is cause and which effect.

34 Harmful immunity: a general scheme

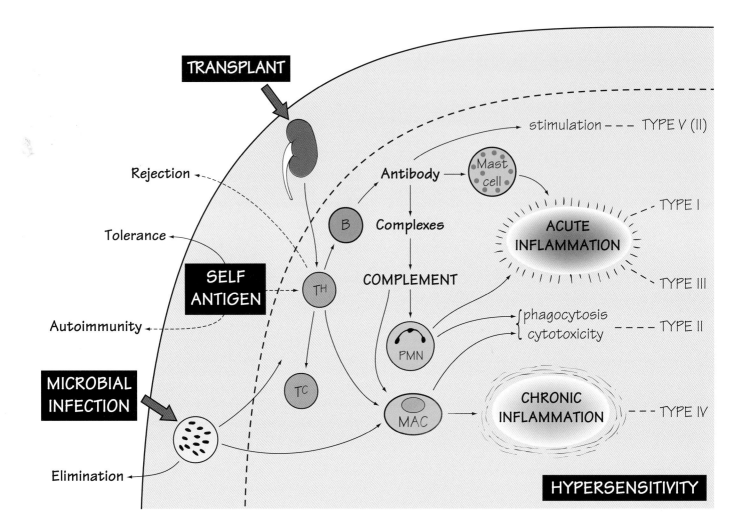

So far we have been considering the successful side of the immune system – its defence role against microbial infection (bottom left). The effectiveness of this is due to two main features: (i) the wide range of pathogens it can specifically recognize and remember, and (ii) the strong non-specific mechanisms it can mobilize to eliminate them.

Unfortunately, both of these abilities can also operate against their possessor.

1 Wide-ranging specificity necessitates an efficient mechanism for avoiding action against 'self' determinants (the problem of **autoimmunity**; centre). Also there are cases where the elimination of non-self material may not be desirable (the problem of **transplant rejection**; top).

2 Strong non-specific weapons (e.g. complement, polymorphs, macrophages and other inflammatory agents; centre) cannot always be trained precisely on the proper target, but may spill over to damage neighbouring tissues (the problem of **hypersensitivity**: right).

The nomenclature of these **immunopathological** reactions has never been very tidy. Originally, any evidence of altered reactivity to

an antigen following prior contact was called 'allergy', while 'hypersensitivity' was defined as 'acute', 'immediate' or 'delayed' on the basis of the time taken for changes – often quite harmless skin test reactions – to appear. In fact 'harmful immunity' can arise as a result of inappropriate or excessive responses to foreign antigens (innocuous ones as in many common allergies and allogeneic transplants or as a by-product of the response to pathogens) or to self antigens (giving rise to autoimmunity). In all these cases the basic mechanisms are often shared and can be usefully classified according to the very influential scheme of Gell and Coombs (extreme right). However, this classification only covers hypersensitivities involving adaptive immunity, and it is becoming increasingly clear that many of the most common degenerative diseases, such as atherosclerosis and Alzheimer's disease are caused by chronic activation of innate immunity, especially macrophages, independently of adaptive immunity. A modified classification that includes 'innate hypersensitivities' is therefore probably needed.

T^H Helper T cell, which by the recognition of carrier determinants permits antibody responses by B cells and the activation of macrophages. T cells recognizing self antigens probably exist in every person but are normally kept in check by a variety of mechanisms (see Figs 22 and 38).

B B lymphocyte, the potential antibody-forming cell. B lymphocytes that recognize many, although probably not all, 'self' determinants are found in normal animals; they can be switched on to make autoantibody by 'part-self' (or 'cross-reacting') antigens if a helper T cell can recognize a 'non-self' determinant on the same antigen (e.g. a drug or a virus; for further details see Fig. 38).

T^C Cytotoxic T cells against 'self' cells have been demonstrated in some autoimmune diseases (e.g. Hashimoto's thyroiditis).

Mast cell A tissue cell with basophilic granules containing vasoactive amines, etc., which can be released following interaction of antigen with passively acquired surface antibody (IgE), resulting in rapid inflammation – local ('allergy') or systemic ('anaphylaxis') (see Fig. 35).

Complexes Combination with antigen is, of course, the basis of all effects of antibody. When there is excess formation of antibody–antigen complexes, some of these settle out of the blood onto the walls of the blood vessels (especially in the skin and kidneys). Tissue damage may then occur from the activation of complement, PMN or platelets (see Fig. 36). Platelet aggregation is a prominent feature of kidney graft rejection. Alternatively, antibodies can form complexes with self antigens on the surface of cells (type II hypersensitivity), activating complement and damaging tissue.

Innate immune damage

Complement is responsible for many of the tissue-damaging effects of antigen–antibody interactions, as well as their useful function against microorganisms. The inflammatory effects are mostly due to the anaphylatoxins (C3a and C5a) which act on mast cells, while opsonization (by C3b) and lysis (by C5–9) are important in the destruction of transplanted cells and (via autoantibody) of autoantigens.

PMN Polymorphonuclear leucocytes are attracted rapidly to sites of inflammation by complement-mediated chemotaxis, where they phagocytose antigen–antibody complexes; their lysosomal enzymes can cause tissue destruction, as in the classic Arthus reaction. Paradoxically, impaired function of these cells such as occurs in chronic granulomatous disease and perhaps also Crohn's disease may lead to chronic bacterial infections becoming established, which in turn lead to chronic inflammation and tissue damage.

MAC Macrophages are important in phagocytosis, but may also be attracted to and activated at the site of antigen persistence, resulting in both tissue necrosis and granuloma formation (see Fig. 37). The slower arrival of monocytes and macrophages in the skin following antigen injection gave rise to the name 'delayed hypersensitivity'. Bacterial lipopolysaccharide (**LPS**) and several other microbial molecules can activate macrophages directly, causing TNF and IL-1 release. When this occurs on a large scale, it can result in vascular collapse and damage to several organs. This 'endotoxin shock' (a type of hypersensitivity of 'innate' immunity) is a feature of infections with meningococci and other Gram-negative bacteria (see Fig. 29). LPS can also directly activate the complement (alternative) and clotting pathways. Macrophages can also be activated by some non-infectious stimuli. Uric acid crystals activate macrophage IL-1 secretion and give rise to the painful symptoms of gout. Chronic macrophage activation by oxidized lipoproteins in blood vessels or the β amyloid protein in brain may underly atherosclerosis and Alzheimer's disease, respectively.

Types of hypersensitivity (Gell and Coombs' classification)

I Acute (allergic; anaphylactic; immediate; reaginic): mediated by IgE antibody together with mast cells (e.g. hay fever). Can also give rise to eosinophil activation, most notably in asthma.

II Antibody mediated (cytotoxic): mediated by IgG or IgM together with complement or phagocytic cells (e.g. blood transfusion reactions, rheumatic fever, many autoimmune diseases).

III Antigen–antibody complex mediated: inflammation involving complement, polymorphs, etc. (e.g. Arthus reaction, serum sickness, SLE, chronic glomerulonephritis).

IV Cell mediated (delayed; tuberculin-type): T-cell dependent recruitment of macrophages, eosinophils, etc. (e.g. tuberculoid leprosy, schistosomal cirrhosis, viral skin rashes, skin graft rejection).

V Stimulatory: a proposal to split off from type II those cases where antibody directly stimulates a cell function (e.g. stimulation of the thyroid TSH receptor in thyrotoxicosis).

35 Allergy and anaphylaxis

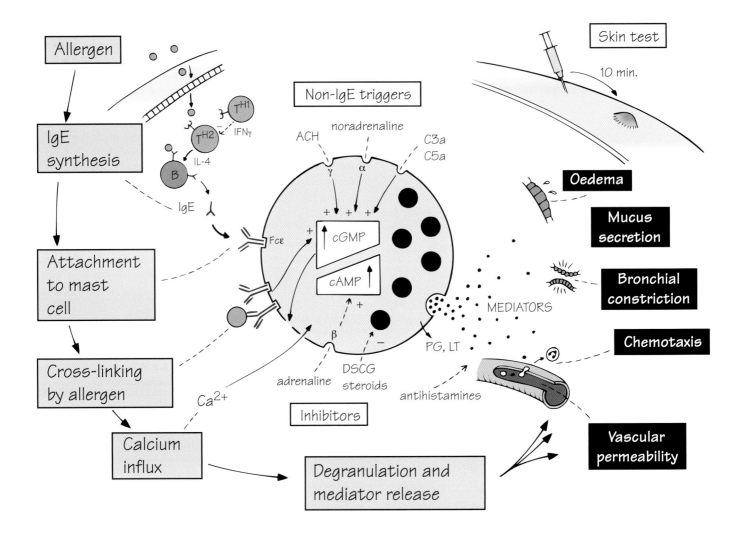

By far the most common form of hypersensitivity is Gell and Coombs' type I, which embraces such everyday **allergic** conditions as hay fever, eczema and urticaria but also the rare and terrifying **anaphylactic** reactions to bee stings, peanuts, penicillin, etc. In both cases the underlying mechanism is a sudden degranulation of **mast cells** (centre) with the release of inflammatory **mediators**, triggered by specific antibodies of the **IgE** class. It is therefore an example of acute inflammation (as already described in Fig. 7) but induced by the presence of a particular antigen rather than by injury or infection. With systemic release (anaphylaxis) there is bronchospasm, vomiting, skin rashes, oedema of the nose and throat, and vascular collapse, sometimes fatal, while with more localized release one or other of these symptoms predominates, depending on the site of exposure to the antigen. Type I hypersensitivity also underlies many cases of asthma, where continuous triggering of local inflammation leads to hypersensitivity of the lung wall and consequent prolonged bronchoconstriction and airway obstruction.

Antigens that can trigger these reactions are known as '**allergens**'. Allergens are often small molecular weight proteins (e.g. insect enzymes) or molecules that bind to host proteins (e.g. penicillins). People who suffer unduly from allergy usually have raised levels of IgE in their blood and are called 'atopic', a trait that is usually inher-

ited, at least 12 genes being involved. As worm antigens are among the most powerful allergens, the existence of this unpleasant and apparently useless form of immune response has been assumed to date from a time when worm infections were a serious evolutionary threat. Inflammation itself, of course, is an invaluable part of the response to injury and infection, and where injury is minimal (e.g. worms in the gut), IgE offers a rapid and specific trigger for increasing access of blood cells, etc. to the area. It is important to note that the term 'allergy' is sometimes used more loosely to describe any adverse response to environmental stimuli, such as allergy to fungal spores experienced by some farmers, which has a totally different immunological basis, or food 'allergies', some of which do not involve the immune system at all.

There is a close link between inflammation and the emotions via the autonomic nervous system, through the influence of the sympathetic (α and β) and parasympathetic (γ) receptors on intracellular levels of the cyclic nucleotides adenosine monophosphate (AMP) and guanosine monophosphate (GMP), which in turn regulate cell function – in the case of mast cells, mediator release (see Fig. 25). Note also that mast cell degranulation can be triggered directly by tissue injury (see Fig. 7) and complement activation (see Fig. 6), and by some bacteria.

IgE The major class of reaginic (skin sensitizing; homocytotropic) antibody. Normally less than 1/10000 of total Ig, its level can be up to 30 times higher, and specific antibody levels 100 times higher, in allergic or worm-infested patients. Binding of its Fc portion to receptors (Fcε) on mast cells and basophils, followed by cross-linking of adjacent molecules by antigen, triggers degranulation. Injection of antigen into the skin of allergic individuals causes inflammation within minutes – the 'immediate skin response'. A humanized monoclonal antibody against IgE (see Fig. 14) has recently been approved for the treatment of severe allergic asthma. IgG antibody, by efficiently removing antigens, can protect against mast cell degranulation.

T^H Helper T cell. IgE production by B cells is dependent on the cytokine IL-4, released by T^{H2} cells. In atopic patients, allergens tend to induce an unbalanced production of the 'T^{H2} type' cytokines IL-4, IL-5, IL-13, etc., but very little of the T^{H1} cytokines such as IFNγ which downregulate IgE production. Drugs that inhibit these cytokines are being tested for treatment of these diseases.

Mast cells in the tissues and blood **basophils** are broadly similar, but there are differences in the content of mediators. There are also important differences between the mast cells in the lung and gut ('mucosal') and those around blood vessels elsewhere ('connective tissue'). Mast cells are regulated by T lymphocytes via cytokine production.

Eosinophils have an important role in inflammation in the lung, which can lead to asthma, and perhaps also to gut inflammatory diseases, including those that may underlie some food allergies. Similar to mast cells they release a variety of inflammatory mediators, and they too are regulated by T-cell-derived cytokines, especially IL-5. They are prominent with PMN, in the 'late phase' reaction that follows up to 24 hours after the immediate response.

Ca^{2+} Following the cross-linking of IgE receptors, membrane lipid changes lead to the entry of calcium, and an increase in adenylate cyclase, which in turn raises cyclic AMP (cAMP) levels.

cAMP, cGMP Cyclic adenosine/guanosine monophosphates, the relative levels of which regulate cell activity. A fall in the cAMP:cGMP ratio is favoured by Ca^{2+} entry and by activation of α and γ receptors, and results in degranulation. Activation of the β receptor (e.g. by adrenaline) has the opposite effect; atopic patients may have a partial defect of β-receptor function, permitting excessive mediator release.

Atopy is a condition characterized by high levels of circulating IgE antibodies, which predisposes the individual to the development of allergy. This is regulated by both genetic and environmental factors, which are currently the object of intense study. The genetic regulation of atopy is complex and multigenic, involving polymorphisms at 20 or more loci. These include polymorphisms in the Fcε receptor, but also non-immunological components such as the receptor for the neurotransmitter 5HT. Interestingly, the prevalence of atopy has increased over the past three decades. This has been variously attributed to increased levels of pollutants in the environment or, more convincingly, to decreased exposure to bacterial infection during early childhood, and hence an imbalance in the developing T^{H1}/T^{H2} balance of the immune system (the so-called hygiene hypothesis).

Asthma is a chronic condition in which the airways become thickened and hypersensitive to environmental stimulation (e.g. during viral infection, or by allergens, dust or even changes in air temperature), which causes them to constrict, resulting in obstruction of the airways and shortness of breath; this can be severe and even fatal. Constriction is thought to be triggered initially by mast cell degranulation (the early phase). Mediators released by the mast cells activate muscle constriction and mucus secretion, but also recruit eosinophils to the lung wall, which in turn degranulate, causing a second delayed episode several hours later. Asthma has a strong genetic predisposition, and there has been an intensive search for gene polymorphisms associated with this disease. Over 25 candidate genes have been identified, and there are probably more. Treatment is still predominantly symptomatic by administering bronchodilators, often delivered by 'inhalers'.

Mediators

Many of these are preformed in the mast cell granules, including **histamine**, which increases vascular permeability and constricts bronchi, **chemotactic** factors for neutrophils and eosinophils, and a factor that activates platelets to release their own mediators. Others are newly formed after the mast cell is triggered, such as prostaglandins (**PG**) and leukotrienes (**LT**; for details see Fig. 7), which have similar effects to histamine but act less rapidly.

Inhibitors

Sodium cromoglycate (**DSCG**; Intal) and **steroids** (e.g. betamethasone) are thought to inhibit mediator release by stabilizing lysosomal membranes. Other drugs used in allergy include **antihistamines** (which do not, however, counteract the other mediators, and are not helpful in asthma); **adrenaline**, isoprenaline, etc., which stimulate β receptors; anticholinergics (e.g. atropine), which block γ receptors; and theophylline, which raises cAMP levels. It has been gratifying to physicians to see the molecular pharmacology of cell regulation confirming so many of their empirical observations on the control of allergic disease.

Non-IgE triggering

The complement products C3a and C5a can cause mast cells to degranulate, and so can some chemicals and insect toxins. Such non-IgE-mediated reactions are called 'anaphylactoid'.

Allergic diseases

The term 'allergy' is often used to cover a whole range of different disorders. Originally, the term 'atopy' referred only to hay fever and asthma, which are usually due to plant or animal 'allergens' in the air, such as pollens, fungi and mites. However, similar allergens may also cause skin reactions (urticaria), either from local contact or following absorption. Urticaria after eating shellfish, strawberries, cows' milk, etc. is a clear case where the site of entry and the site of reaction are quite different, due to the ability of IgE antibodies to attach to mast cells anywhere in the body.

Some allergies do not result from type I hypersensitivity. The allergic reaction of some farmers to hay (farmer's lung) or some individuals to their pets (e.g. pigeon fancier's disease) seem to be due to immune complex formation (type III hypersensitivity). Allergy to wheat gluten (coeliac disease) is probably mediated predominantly by T cells, and may therefore be classified as type IV hypersensitivity. Some food 'allergies', e.g. to milk, do not have an immunological basis at all and are more properly termed 'food intolerance'.

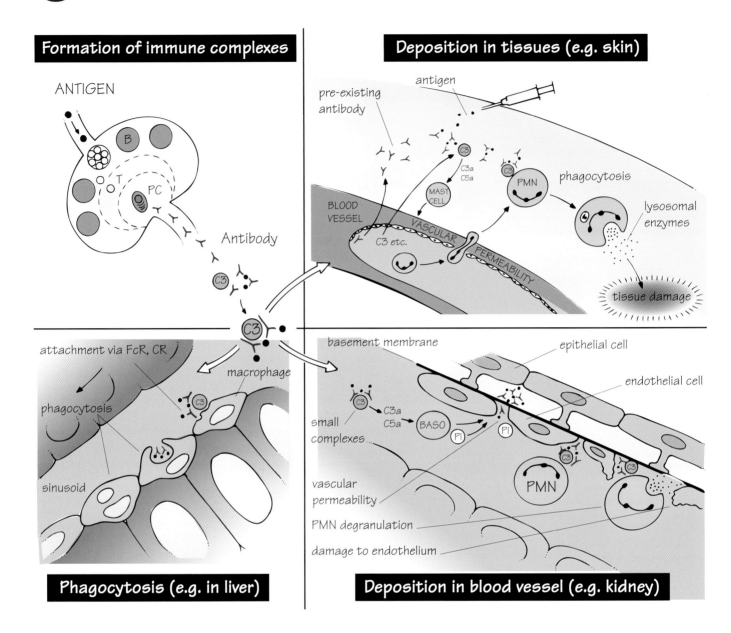

Formation of immune complexes

ANTIGEN

Antibody

Phagocytosis (e.g. in liver)

attachment via FcR, CR

phagocytosis

macrophage

sinusoid

Deposition in tissues (e.g. skin)

antigen

pre-existing antibody

BLOOD VESSEL

VASCULAR PERMEABILITY

C3 etc.

MAST CELL

C3a C5a

PMN

phagocytosis

lysosomal enzymes

tissue damage

Deposition in blood vessel (e.g. kidney)

basement membrane

epithelial cell

endothelial cell

small complexes

C3a C5a

BASO

vascular permeability

PMN degranulation

damage to endothelium

PMN

All the useful functions of antibody depend on its ability to combine with the corresponding antigen to form an **immune complex** (glance back at Fig. 20 to be reminded of the forces that bring this about). The normal fate of these complexes is phagocytosis (bottom left), which is greatly enhanced if complement becomes attached to the complex; thus, complex formation is an essential prelude to antigen disposal.

However, there are circumstances when this fails to happen, particularly if the complexes are small (e.g. with proportions such as Ag2:Ab1 or Ag3:Ab2). This can occur if there is an **excess** of antigen, as in persistent infections and in autoimmunity, where the antibody is of very low affinity or where there are defects of the phagocytic or the complement systems.

If not rapidly phagocytosed, complexes can induce serious inflammatory changes in either the tissues (top right) or in the walls of small blood vessels (bottom right), depending on the site of formation. In both cases it is activation of **complement** and enzyme release by **polymorphs** that do the damage. The renal glomerular capillaries are particularly vulnerable, and immune complex disease is the most common cause of chronic glomerulonephritis, which is itself the most frequent cause of kidney failure.

Note that increased vascular permeability plays a preparatory role both for complex deposition in vessels and for exudation of complement and PMN into the tissues, underlining the close links between type I and type III hypersensitivity. Likewise there is an overlap with type II, in that some cases of glomerulonephritis are caused by antibody against the basement membrane itself, but produce virtually identical damage.

Complexes of small size are formed in antigen excess, as occurs early in the antibody response to a large dose of antigen, or with persistent exposure to drugs or chronic infections (e.g. streptococci, hepatitis, malaria), or associated with autoantibodies.

Fc receptors (FcR) A family of receptors found at the surface of many cell types that bind to the constant (known historically as the Fc) region of antibodies (see Fig. 14). Fc receptors on macrophages and neutrophils facilitate phagocytosis, and are responsible for the opsonizing effects of antibody. Most Fc receptors bind much more efficiently to antibodies that form part of an antigen–antibody complex, thus ensuring that free antibody in serum does not fill up the receptors and interfere with their function.

PC Plasma cells are the last stage of differentiation of activated B cells. Plasma cells are long-lived cells that settle in the medulla of lymph nodes, or in the bone marrow, and produce extraordinarily large amounts of specific antibody until they die.

Macrophages lining the liver (Kupffer cells) or spleen sinusoids remove particles from the blood, including large complexes.

PMN Polymorphonuclear leucocyte, the principal phagocyte of blood, with granules (lysosomes) that contain numerous antibacterial enzymes. When these are released neighbouring cells are often damaged. This is particularly likely to happen when PMNs attempt to phagocytose complexes that are fixed to other tissues.

C3 The central component of complement, a series of serum proteins involved in inflammation and antibacterial immunity. When complexes bind C1, C4 and C2, C3 is split into a small fragment, C3a, which activates mast cells and basophils, and a larger one, C3b, which promotes phagocytosis by attaching to receptors on PMNs and macrophages (CR in figure). Subsequent components generate chemotactic factors that attract PMNs to the site. C3 can also be split via the 'alternative' pathway initiated by bacterial endotoxins, etc. Complement is also responsible for preventing the formation of large precipitates and solubilizing precipitates once they have formed (see also Fig. 6).

Mast cells, **basophils**, and **platelets** contribute to increased vascular permeability by releasing histamine, etc. (see Fig. 35).

The **glomerular basement membrane** (GBM), together with endothelial cells and external epithelial 'podocytes', separates blood from urine. Immune complexes are usually trapped on the blood side of the basement membrane, except when antibody is directed specifically against the GBM itself (as in the autoimmune disease Goodpasture's syndrome) but small complexes can pass through the basement membrane to accumulate in the urinary space. Mesangial cells may proliferate into the subendothelial space, presumably in an attempt to remove complexes. Endothelial proliferation may occur too, resulting in glomerular thickening and loss of function.

Immune complex diseases
The classic types of immune complex disease, neither of which is much seen nowadays, are the Arthus reaction, in which antigen injected into the skin of animals with high levels of antibody induces local tissue necrosis (top right in figure), and serum sickness, in which passively injected serum, e.g. a horse antiserum used to treat pneumonia, induces an antibody response, early in the course of which small complexes are deposited in various blood vessels, causing a fever with skin and joint

symptoms about a week later. However, certain diseases are thought to represent essentially the same type of pathological reactions.

SLE Systemic lupus erythematosus, a disease of unknown origin in which autoantibodies to nuclear antigens (which include DNA, RNA and DNA/RNA-associated proteins) are deposited, with complement, in the kidney, skin, joints, brain, etc. The immune complexes also stimulate plasmacytoid dendritic cells to produce very high levels of type I interferons which contribute to inflammation (see Fig. 24). Treatment is by immunosuppression or, in severe cases, exchange transfusion to deplete autoantibody.

Polyarteritis nodosa An inflammatory disease of small arteries affecting numerous organs. Some cases may be due to complexes of hepatitis B antigen with antibody and complement.

RA Rheumatoid arthritis features both local (Arthus-type) damage to joint surfaces and systemic vasculitis. The cause is unknown but complexes between autoantibodies and IgG (rheumatoid factor) are a constant finding. Immune complexes bind to macrophages within joints inducing the release of tumour necrosis fact (see Fig. 24) and RA in many patients can be effectively treated by administering antibodies to TNF-α. The symptoms of RA are also alleviated by removing circulating B cells by administering an antibody to the B-cell marker CD20.

Alveolitis caused by *Actinomyces* and other fungi (see Fig. 30) may be due to an Arthus-type reaction in the lung (e.g. farmer's lung). Similar immune complex disease reactions occur in some individuals who keep pigeons or other birds.

Thyroiditis, Goodpasture's syndrome, and other autoimmune diseases can be caused by antibodies binding to 'self' antigens on these tissues (a 'type II' hypersensitivity reaction), hence causing damage to the organ.

Infectious diseases The skin rashes, joint pains and renal complications of several infections can be caused by type III reactions. Very high levels of antibody (most of it non-specific) are also associated with some parasitic diseases such as malaria. In addition, widespread activation of complement can occur in septic shock, induced by LPS from Gram-negative bacteria, and in the haemorrhagic shock of viruses such as dengue, in both of which it is associated with cytokines such as TNF. Complement, neutrophils and cytokines are also thought to be involved in the pulmonary vascular leakage of the adult respiratory distress syndrome (ARDS) that follows massive trauma.

Haemolytic disease of the newborn
In general, mothers are tolerant to the antigens carried by their fetus. However, women who do not carry the red blood cell Rhesus antigen D (Rh negative) can sometimes become immunized against this antigen by a Rh-positive fetus at birth, when blood cells of the fetus can enter the mother's circulation due to damage to the placenta. The antibodies cross the placenta in a subsequent pregnancy and cause serious anaemia in the fetus. This danger can be substantially reduced by administering anti-Rh antibodies to the mother at the time of birth, thus rapidly removing the circulating fetal blood cells from the mother's circulation and preventing the initial immunization.

Note that this is not really an immune complex disease, but would be classified as Gell and Coombs' type II.

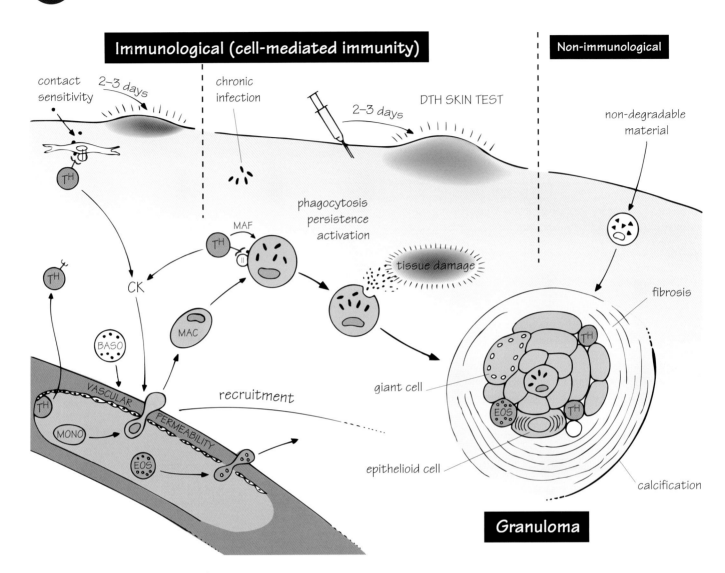

Following the changes in permeability, the activation of complement and the influx of polymorphs, the last arrivals at sites of inflammation are the 'mononuclear cells': **lymphocytes** and **monocytes** (bottom left). Lymphocytes are usually specific in their attack, and only cause harm when attack is not called for (i.e. when the target is 'self' or a transplant), but monocytes and macrophages are equipped with enzymes that they normally use in the process of mopping up dead tissue cells and polymorphs, but which can also damage healthy cells, including other macrophages. When the stimulus is persistent, the result may be a growing mass of macrophages, or granuloma (bottom right), the hallmark of **chronic inflammation**.

These changes can occur in the absence of any specific immune response (e.g. reactions to foreign bodies; top right), but they are often greatly augmented by the activity of specific T lymphocytes (left) which, by secreting cytokines, attract and immobilize monocytes and activate macrophages. When this process is predominantly beneficial (as in healed tuberculosis) we speak of '**cell-mediated immunity**' (CMI); when it is harmful (as in contact sensitivity or schistosomal cirrhosis) it is termed '**type IV hypersensitivity**', the underlying mechanism being the same and the difference one of emphasis (compare with Fig. 21). Confusingly, direct killing by cytotoxic T cells is also called 'cell-mediated immunity', although because it mainly affects virus-containing cells, a better name would be 'cell-mediated autoimmunity' or, in the case of organ grafts, 'cell-mediated transplant rejection'.

In any case, it is rare for one type of tissue damage to occur in isolation, interaction of cells and sharing of biochemical pathways being a feature of immune mechanisms, useful and harmful alike.

Cell-mediated immunity (CMI) Contact between recirculating T cells and antigen leads to cytokine secretion with attraction and activation of monocytes and other myeloid cells (for further details see Fig. 21). In the case of persistent antigens, particularly with intracellular infections such as tuberculosis, leprosy, brucellosis, leishmaniasis, schistosomiasis (the egg granuloma), trichinosis and fungi such as *Histoplasma* spp., chronic inflammation may result. The principal cell type associated with CMI has long been thought to be the T^{H1} cell, via the release of IFNγ and other macrophage activating factors. However, more recently, attention has focused on the T^{17} cell (see Fig. 21), which seems to play a key part in mediating tissue damage in several infectious and autoimmune diseases, principally via recruitment of granulocytes.

Delayed-type hypersensitivity (DTH) One of the key features of CMI, antigen-specific memory, can be tested *in vitro* by measuring lymphocyte proliferation or the release of cytokines such as IFNγ, or *in vivo* by the response to antigen injected into the skin. A positive DTH response consists of a reddened swelling 2–3 days later, the Mantoux or Heaf tests for tuberculosis being typical examples. While DTH frequently correlates with protective immunity, this is not invariably the case. Sometimes basophils are prominent, giving a quicker response known as 'Jones Mote' hypersensitivity.

Contact sensitivity In this variant of DTH, antigens (usually plant or chemical molecules) react with proteins in the skin and stimulate a T^H and T^C cell response. The result is an eczema-like reaction with oedema and mononuclear cell infiltration 1–2 days later. Contact sensitivity to nickel in watches or jewellery is one of the most common forms of contact allergic dermatitis.

Chronic non-immunological inflammation Materials that are phagocytosed but cannot be degraded, or that are toxic to macrophages, such as talc, silica, asbestos, and the cell wall peptidoglycan of group A streptococci, will give rise to granulomas even in T-cell-deprived animals, and are therefore considered to be able to activate macrophages without the aid of T cells. A number of chronic degenerative diseases (e.g Alzheimer's disease in brain, and atherosclerosis in vessels) are associated with T-independent macrophage inflammatory responses, although it remains unclear whether the inflammatory response is a primary cause of disease, or a secondary response to some other underlying pathology. The controversial reports that antioxidants increase lifespan may perhaps be due to their ability to dampen down macrophage-mediated tissue damage.

Cancer Chronic inflammation associated with infection is strongly associated with the development of cancer. Examples include *Helicobacter pylori*, which gives rises to ulcers and strongly increases the risk of developing stomach cancer. Similarly, chronic infection with hepatitis B or C viruses often leads to liver cancer. The mechanisms that link inflammation and cancer include increased angiogenesis, the formation of new blood vessels that provide nutrients and oxygen for tumour cells to grow.

Granulomas

Granulomas, aggregates of macrophages, lymphocytes, and a variety of other cell types, are an important feature of several chronic infections, most notably tuberculosis. They are initiated and maintained principally by the recruitment of macrophages by T cells into a site of persistent antigen or toxic material. Immune complexes are also a stimulus for granuloma formation.

Tissue damage within a granuloma is caused principally by lysosomal enzymes released by macrophages, and by reactive oxygen species produced by the oxidative burst (see Fig. 9). The centre of older granulomas therefore often consists of necrotic (dying) tissue. However, as granulomas grow, they frequently damage the surrounding organ, e.g. by obstructing and rupturing blood vessels, or airways in the lung in tuberculosis.

Epithelioid cells are large cells found in palisades around areas of necrotic tissue. They are thought to derive from macrophages, specialized for enzyme secretion rather than phagocytosis.

Giant cells are formed by fusion of macrophages; they are particularly prominent in 'foreign-body' granulomas.

Eosinophils are often found in granulomas, perhaps attracted by antigen–antibody complexes, but also under the influence of T cells.

Fibrosis around a granuloma represents an attempt at 'healing'. Long-standing granulomas, e.g. healed tuberculosis, may eventually calcify, e.g. the well-known Ghon focus in the lung X-ray of many healthy people.

Granulomatous diseases

Granulomas are found in several diseases, some of known and some of unknown aetiology, suggesting an irritant or immunological origin. A few of the better known are listed below.

Sarcoidosis is characterized by granulomas in the lung, skin, eye, etc. An interesting but paradoxical feature is a profound deficiency of other cell-mediated T-cell immunity (e.g. a loss of Mantoux test responses) and often an increased Ig level and antibody responsiveness.

Crohn's disease (regional ileitis) is somewhat similar to sarcoidosis, but usually restricted to the intestine. It is associated with pronounced T-cell infiltration into the intestinal wall, and hence was thought to be due to autoimmunity against gut proteins, perhaps stimulated by cross-reacting bacteria. However, Crohn's disease is associated with a genetic defect in the bacterial-sensing NOD proteins (see Fig. 5), and may be more similar to **chronic granulomatous disease** in deriving from a failure to effectively clear chronic bacterial infection from the gut. **Ulcerative colitis** may have a similar aetiology.

Temporal arteritis is a chronic inflammatory disease of arteries, with granulomas in which giant cells are prominent.

Primary biliary cirrhosis In this rare autoimmune disease (see also Fig. 38), granulomas form around the bile ducts. The disease is believed to result from cross-reaction between a bacterial antigen and a mitochondrial 'self antigen'.

Eosinophilic granuloma Sometimes eosinophils outnumber the other cells in a granuloma; this is particularly seen in worm infections and in rare bone conditions.

Chronic granulomatous disease (CGD) An immunodeficiency disease, characterized by a defect in granulocyte function, which leads to chronic bacterial infection and granuloma development (see Fig. 33).

38 Autoimmune disease

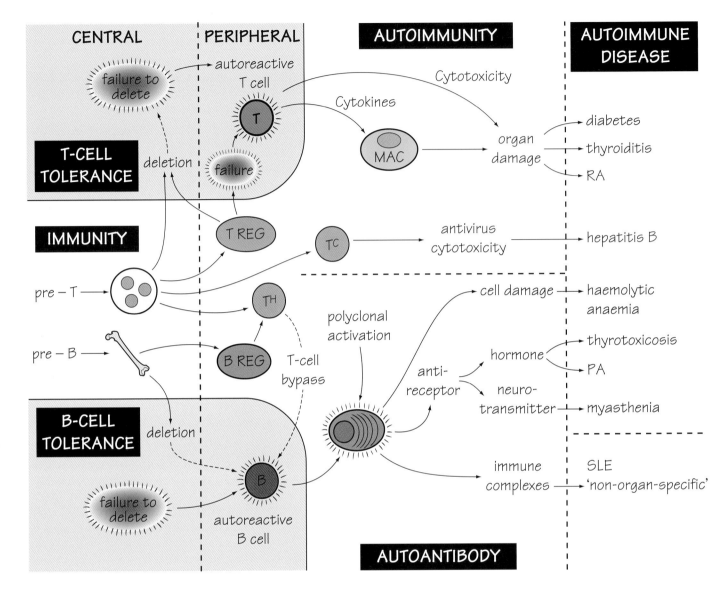

Autoimmunity represents the failure of self-tolerance. Before proceeding, the reader is recommended to glance back at Fig. 22, which summarizes the mechanisms by which the immune system normally safeguards its lymphocytes against self-reactivity. This is essentially a problem for the adaptive immune system, since both B and T cells generate their antigen-binding receptors by random gene rearrangement (see Figs 12 and 13) and receptors recognizing self antigens are bound to be generated in the process.

The main mechanisms by which these are prevented from causing harm are shown in Fig. 22. The figure above highlights some of the points at which they can break down or be induced to fail. These are numerous, but two influences are particularly significant: *genetics* and *infection*. Identical twins show concordance rates around 30% for many autoimmune diseases (concordance is the frequency of disease in one twin occurring in the other). The association of autoimmune diseases with individual HLA genes, especially class II, implies a crucial role for CD4+ T cells, although the association is fairly weak

(relative risk 4–14; relative risk is the chance of developing the disease compared with people without the gene) except for ankylosing spondylitis, where the very strong link (over 90) is with a class I gene, B 27. The role of infection in autoimmunity is suggestive but seldom clear-cut: autoimmune disease frequently follows infection, but no autoimmune disease has been convincingly shown to be due to a specific pathogen. The killing of virus-infected cells by cytotoxic T cells could be regarded as an exception, but here the autodestruction is a beneficial part of recovery, although it may cause excessive damage, e.g. hepatitis B and the myocarditis of coxsackie virus infection.

It is important to realize that **autoimmunity** (centre of figure) does not necessarily mean **autoimmune disease** (right), the latter term being restricted to conditions where there is reasonable evidence that the symptoms are in fact due to autoantibodies and/or autoreactive T cells (see opposite page). The finding of autoantibodies in the absence of obvious disease, or even in healthy people, emphasizes the fact that the precise aetiology of most autoimmune diseases is still not fully understood.

Self-tolerance and self-reactivity

Tolerance The mechanisms responsible for making sure that lymphocytes do not generally react to self antigens (self-tolerance) are explored in Fig. 22. However, in some cases tolerance is not complete. This can result from incomplete clonal deletion, or a breakdown in peripheral tolerance. Deficiency in the T^{REG} subpopulation has been reported in several autoimmune diseases, including diabetes, rheumatoid arthritis and SLE. Expression of class II MHC antigens on thyroid epithelial cells, or pancreatic beta cells, perhaps as a result of infection, may also contribute to breakdown of tolerance. Sometimes, tissue injury or infection can allow antigens that are usually screened from the immune system (e.g. in the eye) to become accessible.

Macrophages have a key role in many autoimmune diseases, by releasing cytokines that cause local inflammation, enzymes and reactive chemicals (free radicals) that damage the tissue. Antibodies against TNF-α, a key macrophage-derived inflammatory cytokine, are very effective in treatment of rheumatoid arthritis, psoriasis and Crohn's disease. Macrophage activation is dependent on autoreactive T^H cells that release IFNγ and IL-17.

Cytotoxic T cells (T^C) in killing virus-infected cells, may damage normal tissues. Liver damage in hepatitis B is a classic example. In other cases, however, autoreactive T^C 'break tolerance' and target specific autoantigens in organs such as the thyroid or the pancreas.

Drugs frequently bind to blood cells, either directly (e.g. sedormid to platelets; penicillin to red cells) or as complexes with antibody (e.g. quinidine). Alpha methyldopa can induce antibodies against Rhesus blood group antigens, towards which B-cell tolerance is particularly unstable.

Cross-reacting antigens shared between microbe and host may stimulate T help for otherwise silent self-reactive B cells – the 'T-cell bypass'. Cardiac damage in streptococcal infections and Chagas' disease appear to be examples of this.

Polyclonal activation Many microbial products (e.g. endotoxins, DNA) can stimulate B cells, including self-reactive ones. The EB virus infects B cells themselves and can make them proliferate continuously.

Autoantibodies are found in every individual but rarely cause disease. In some diseases, raised autoantibody levels are clearly effect rather than cause (e.g. cardiolipin antibodies in syphilis). But in some diseases they are the first, major or only detectable abnormality and can cause damage in a variety of ways. They can attach to tissues and activate the complement system (see Fig. 6) leading to inflammation. They can react with specific receptors blocking important hormone or neurotransmitter signals. Or they can react with target autoantigens in blood, forming large complexes (see Figs 20 and 36), which accumulate in skin, lung or kidneys causing inflammation and organ damage.

Autoimmune diseases

The precise mechanisms that give rise to autoimmune diseases remain incompletely understood. Much of our current knowledge comes from the study of animal models, such as experimental allergic encephalitis and collagen-induced arthritis, in which autoimmunity is induced by direct immunization with self-proteins. These models have taught us much about how tolerance may be broken, but important differences remain between the corresponding animal and human diseases.

Genetics of autoimmunity Most autoimmune diseases have a genetic component and much effort is being devoted to identifying the genetic 'risk factors' associated with particular autoimmune diseases. The strongest associations are those with specific alleles of the MHC class II genes (see opposite page), confirming that CD4+ T cells have an important role in the aetiology of these diseases. However, there are at least 20 other loci that contribute to an individual's propensity to develop a particular autoimmune disease. Some of these appear to control the level of cytokines, others affect signalling pathways in immune cells while yet others affect non-immunological steps in tissue damage.

Haemolytic anaemia and *thrombocytopenia,* although they can be caused by drugs, are more often idiopathic. The correlation between autoantibody levels and red cell destruction is not always very close, suggesting another pathological process at work.

Thyroiditis is one of the best candidates for 'primary' autoimmunity. There may be stimulation (thyrotoxicosis) by antibody against the receptor for pituitary TSH, or inhibition (myxoedema) by cell destruction, probably mediated by cytotoxic T cells and autoantibody.

Pernicious anaemia results from a deficiency of gastric intrinsic factor, the normal carrier for vitamin B_{12}. This can be caused both by autoimmune destruction of the parietal cells (atrophic gastritis) and by autoantibodies to intrinsic factor itself.

Diabetes, Addison's disease (adrenal hypofunction) and other endocrine diseases are often found together in patients or families, suggesting an underlying genetic predisposition. The actual damage is probably mainly T-cell mediated, against pancreatic β cells and the adrenal cortex, respectively.

Myasthenia gravis, in which neuromuscular transmission is intermittently defective, is associated with autoantibodies to, and destruction of, the postsynaptic acetylcholine receptors. There are often thymic abnormalities and thymectomy may be curative, although it is not really clear why.

Rheumatoid arthritis is characterized by autoantibody against IgG (rheumatoid factor) although not in every case. Joint damage may be partly mediated via immune complexes, and injections of antibodies against CD20, which result in depletion of B cells, is an effective treatment in a proportion of patients. T-cell-dependent activation of macrophages (type IV hypersensitivity) may also contribute. In either case the cytokines TNF-α and IL-1 cause the main pathology, by activating degradation of cartilage.

SLE In systemic lupus erythematosus the autoantibodies are against nuclear antigens, including DNA, RNA and nucleic acid binding proteins. The resulting immune complex deposition is widespread throughout the vascular system, giving rise to a 'non-organ-specific' pattern of disease. A localizing role for the antigen itself may explain why different complexes damage different organs. Patients with SLE also have very high levels of type I interferons, perhaps resulting from innate responses to circulating nucleic acids (see Fig. 5), which contribute to a generalized inflammation.

Treatment of autoimmunity

No cures exist for most autoimmune diseases, and treatment is symptomatic; examples are anti-inflammatory drugs for rheumatoid arthritis, insulin for type I diabetes, anti-thyroid drugs for thyrotoxicosis. Where autoantibodies are to blame (e.g. in myasthenia) plasmapheresis to remove them can provide short-term benefit. Remarkable improvement in patients with rheumatoid arthritis and Crohn's disease has been achieved by treatment with a high-affinity antibody against TNF-α, which presumably blocks the inflammatory cascade within the affected tissue: this remains the best example of successful therapy using an anticytokine antibody. More antigen-specific approaches to immunomodulation, such as vaccination against particular families of T-cell receptors, or the simulation of specific T^{REG} cells, are still at an experimental stage.

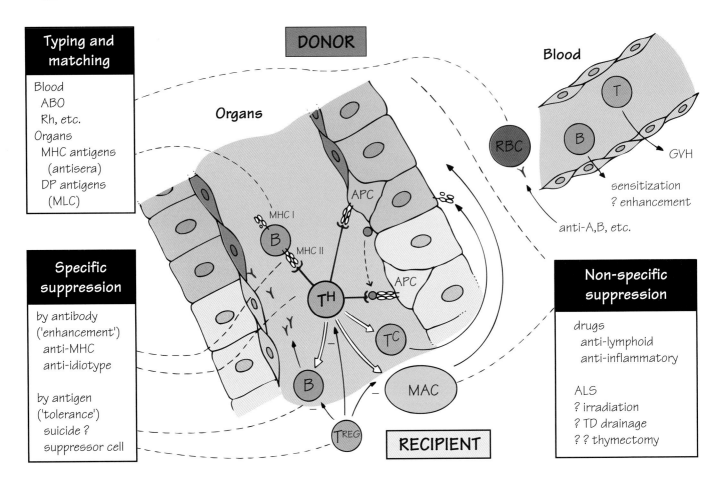

Typing and matching

Blood
  ABO
  Rh, etc.
Organs
  MHC antigens
    (antisera)
  DP antigens
    (MLC)

Specific suppression

by antibody
  ('enhancement')
  anti-MHC
  anti-idiotype

by antigen
  ('tolerance')
  suicide ?
  suppressor cell

Non-specific suppression

drugs
  anti-lymphoid
  anti-inflammatory

ALS
? irradiation
? TD drainage
? ? thymectomy

The success of organ grafts between identical ('syngeneic'*) twins, and their rejection in all other cases, reflects the remarkable strength of immunological recognition of cell-surface antigens within a species. This is an unfortunate (and in the evolutionary sense unforeseeable) result of the specialization of T cells for detecting **alterations of MHC antigens**, upon which all adaptive responses depend (for a reminder of the central role of T-helper cells see Figs 19 and 21), plus the enormous degree of **MHC polymorphism** (different antigens in different individuals; see Fig. 11). It appears that when confronted with 'non-self' MHC molecules, T cells confuse them with 'self plus antigen', and in most cases probably 'self plus virus'; several clear examples of this have already been found in mouse experiments. This may be one of the reasons for MHC polymorphism itself: the more different varieties of 'self' a species contains, the less likely is any particular virus to pass undetected and decimate the whole species. Differences in red cell ('blood group') antigens also give trouble in blood transfu-

sion (top right) because of antibody; here the rationale for polymorphism is less obvious, but it is much more restricted (e.g. six ABO phenotypes compared with over 10^{12} for MHC). The 'minor' histocompatibility and blood group antigens appear to be both less polymorphic and antigenically weaker.

Graft rejection can be mediated by T and/or B cells, with their usual non-specific effector adjuncts (complement, cytotoxic cells, macrophages, etc.), depending on the target: antibody destroys cells free in the blood, and reacts with vascular endothelium (e.g. of a grafted organ; centre) to initiate type II or III hypersensitivity, while T cells attack solid tissue directly or via macrophages (type IV). Unless the recipient is already sensitized to donor antigens, these processes do not take effect for a week or more, confirming that rejection is due to adaptive, not innate, immunity.

Successful organ grafting relies at present on (top left) matching donor and recipient MHC antigens as far as possible (relatives and especially siblings are more likely to share these), and (bottom right) suppressing the residual immune response. The ideal would be (bottom left) to induce specific unresponsiveness to MHC antigens, but this is still experimental (see Fig. 40).

*Terminology: auto, same individual; syngeneic, syngraft, between genetically identical individuals; allo, non-identical, within species; xeno, between species.

Typing and matching

For blood transfusion, the principle is simple: **A** and/or **B** antigens are detected by agglutination with specific antisera; this is always necessary because normal individuals have antibody against whichever antigen they lack. **Rh** (Rhesus) antigens are also typed to avoid sensitizing women to those that a prospective child might carry, as Rh incompatibility can cause serious haemolytic disease in the fetus. Minor antigens only cause trouble in patients sensitized by repeated transfusions. Other possible consequences of blood transfusion are **sensitization** against MHC antigens carried on B cells and, in severely immunodeficient patients, **GVH** (graft-versus-host) reactions by transfused T cells against host antigens. The latter is a major complication of bone-marrow grafting.

For organ (e.g. kidney) grafting, MHC antigens must be typed by DNA typing, in which haplotype is determined using polymerase chain reaction (PCR) and allele-specific pairs of primers. The success of kidney grafting is related to the degree of match, particularly class II (DR), although the better results with relatives suggest that there are other 'minor' histocompatibility loci, which are still being identified.

Rejection

The initial event is the recognition of 'altered self' class II antigens by T-helper cells. This can occur either by direct contact with donor B cells or antigen-presenting cells (light green APC in figure) or via the uptake of soluble donor antigens (shaded circles) by the recipient's own APC (darker green). After this, B cells, cytotoxic T cells and macrophages are all triggered into action, which response destroys the graft depends on the organ in question. Some points of special interest are listed below.

Kidney graft rejection can be **immediate**, due to ABO mismatch or pre-existing anti HLA antibodies, **acute** (weeks to months) due to the immune response or **chronic** (months to years) due to repeated minor rejection episodes or re-emergence of immune complex-mediated disease. Surprisingly, blood transfusion before grafting improves survival, perhaps by inducing enhancing antibodies against class II donor antigens. Immunosuppression has improved transplant success to over 70%, principally by decreasing the occurrence of acute rejection. The causes of chronic rejection, in contrast, remain poorly understood.

Bone marrow contains the haemopoietic stem cell, and is therefore required whenever it is necessary to replace the host haemopoietic system (e.g. in some immunodeficiencies or after high-dose chemotherapy). The growth factor G-CSF causes haemopoietic stem cells to come out of the bone marrow and enter the circulation. As a result, blood can be used in place of bone marrow, a procedure known as peripheral stem cell transplantation. Any haemopoietic grafts are vigorously rejected, and require strong immunosuppression. In addition, they can kill the host by GVH reaction, unless T cells are removed from the donor marrow. In some cases GVH by the graft can help to kill the original tumour cells (graft-versus-tumour [GVT]), but balancing GVT and GVH remains a difficult clinical challenge.

Liver grafts are not so strongly rejected, and may even induce a degree of tolerance. HLA typing is less important. Sometimes, temporary organ transplants may be sufficient. In a recent example, a boy whose liver was damaged by a virus infection received adult liver cells coated with a chemical found in algae which prevented them from being attacked by the immune system. The donor cells survived a few months, long enough for the recipient's liver to recover normal function.

Endocrine organs survive unexpectedly well if cultured or otherwise treated to remove the minority of cells expressing class II antigens.

Skin grafts are rejected very vigorously by T cells, perhaps because of their extensive vascularization. For this reason, skin transplantation is usually autologous or a temporary graft is used to protect the underlying tissue while the host's own skin regenerates (e.g. after extensive burns).

Cornea and *cartilage,* being non-vascular tissues (immune privileged sites), are less accessible to the immune system. Nevertheless, corneas are rejected in about 25% of cases, although the mechanisms leading to graft recognition remain unclear.

The normal *fetus* is of course an allograft, and why it is not rejected is still something of a mystery, despite evidence for a number of possible mechanisms, including specific suppressor cells, serum blocking and immunosuppressive factors, and special properties of both placenta (maternal) and trophoblast (fetal).

Xenografts There is considerable interest in the possibility of using pigs as animal donors for organ transplantation because of the continuing shortfall of available human organs. However, pig xenografts are rejected in primates within minutes by a process of hyperacute rejection. This is due to a combination of preformed antibodies against carbohydrate structures found in pigs but not primates, and the fact that the complement-regulating proteins on pig tissue (e.g. DAF; see Fig. 6) do not interact well with human complement. There is also continuing concern that pigs may harbour novel retroviruses, which could 'jump' the species barrier during transplantation and cause a new epidemic similar to AIDS.

Organ cloning Because of the continual shortage of donors for organ transplants, there is enormous excitement about the possibility of growing 'designer' organs by differentiating stem cells (whether embryonic or non-embryonic) in culture. There has been great progress towards achieving this remarkable technical feat in animal models. However, as embryonic stem cells will generally be derived from a different individual than the organ recipient, the question of immunological rejection remains.

Immunosuppression (for further details see Fig. 40)

Non-specific The success of modern transplantation surgery is due largely to the introduction of cyclosporin, and later FK506, two drugs that selectively block the activation of T cells in an antigen non-specific way (see Fig. 12). These two drugs, together with some cytotoxic drugs, are used at high concentrations postoperatively to block the initial acute rejection, and then at lower maintenance doses to block chronic rejection. Some other approaches are shown in Fig. 40.

Specific suppression is directed at either the antigens inducing a response or the receptors on the cells carrying it out. When brought about by antibody, this is conventionally called **enhancement** and when by antigen, **tolerance**. Antigen-specific suppression is the goal of transplantation immunologists, but has still to be demonstrated in humans.

Regulatory T cells (T^{REG}) can suppress ongoing immune responses in an antigen-specific way (see Fig. 22). Isolating and expanding T^{REG} cells in culture and then reintroducing them into a graft recipient has shown considerable promise in preventing rejection in animal models, and ways to translate this into clinical treatments are being actively pursued.

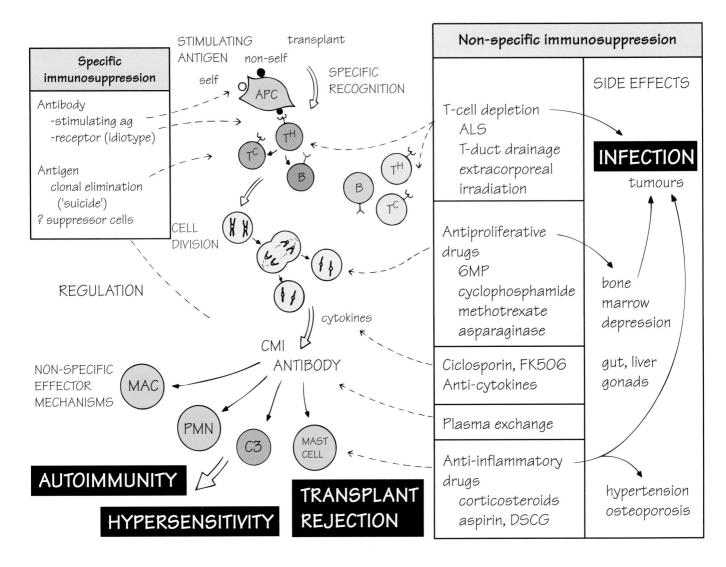

Specific immunosuppression

Antibody
  -stimulating ag
  -receptor (idiotype)
 	
Antigen
  clonal elimination
    ('suicide')
? suppressor cells

STIMULATING ANTIGEN
transplant
non-self
self
SPECIFIC RECOGNITION
APC
T^H
T^C
B
CELL DIVISION
REGULATION
cytokines
CMI
ANTIBODY
NON-SPECIFIC EFFECTOR MECHANISMS
MAC
PMN
C3
MAST CELL

AUTOIMMUNITY

HYPERSENSITIVITY

TRANSPLANT REJECTION

Non-specific immunosuppression	
	SIDE EFFECTS

T-cell depletion
  ALS
  T-duct drainage
  extracorporeal
  irradiation
	INFECTION
	tumours

Antiproliferative drugs
  6MP
  cyclophosphamide
  methotrexate
  asparaginase
	bone marrow depression

Ciclosporin, FK506 Anti-cytokines	gut, liver gonads
Plasma exchange	

Anti-inflammatory drugs
  corticosteroids
  aspirin, DSCG
	hypertension osteoporosis

Suppression of immune responses, a regular part of the management of organ transplantation, can also be of value in cases of severe hypersensitivity and autoimmunity. Most of the methods currently available are more or less non-specific, and their use is limited by dangerous side-effects (right).

The problem is to interfere with specific T and/or B cells (top centre, darker colour) or their effects, without causing damage to other vital functions. T cells can be **depleted** by antilymphocyte antisera (ALS) and by removing or damaging recirculating cells (which are mostly T); however, this will remove not only undesirable lymphocytes, but also others upon whose normal response to infection life may depend (**B**, **T**, lighter colour). Lymphocytes almost always divide in the course of responding to antigen (centre), so drugs that inhibit **cell division** are effective immunosuppressants (the same drugs tend to be useful in treating cancer for the same reason); here the danger is that other dividing tissues, such as bone marrow and intestinal epithelium, will also be inhibited. A third point of attack is the **non-specific effector mechanisms** involved in the 'inflammatory' pathways (bottom) which so often cause the actual damage, but here again useful and harmful elements are knocked out indiscriminately.

What is clearly needed is an attack focused on antigen-specific lymphocytes, i.e. an attack via their receptors (top left). This might take the form of masking the antigens by which they are stimulated, masking or removing the receptors themselves, or using them to deliver a 'suicidal' dose of antigen to the cell. Whether any of these experimental approaches will be effective enough to replace the present clumsy but well-tried methods of immunosuppression time will tell.

Non-specific immunosuppression

ALS (antilymphocyte serum) is made by immunizing horses or rabbits with human lymphocytes and absorbing out unwanted specificities. It depletes especially T cells, probably largely by opsonizing them for phagocytosis. It has found a limited use in organ transplantation. Monoclonal antibodies to B cells, particularly to CD20 on the B-cell surface, were originally introduced to treat B-cell lymphomas (see Fig. 42), but have also proved useful in treatment of rheumatoid arthritis. Antibodies to particular T-cell subsets or surface molecules, such as CD4, may have a more useful future.

Extracorporeal irradiation of blood, and **thoracic duct drainage** are drastic measures to deplete recirculating T cells, occasionally used in transplant rejection crises.

6MP (6-mercaptopurine) and its precursor **azathioprine** (Imuran) block purine metabolism, which is needed for DNA synthesis; despite side effects on bone marrow polymorph and platelet production, they were for many years standard therapy in organ transplantation and widely used in autoimmune diseases, e.g. rheumatoid arthritis and SLE. A more recent analogue is mycophenolate mofetil.

Cyclophosphamide and *chlorambucil* are 'alkylating' agents, which cross-link DNA strands and prevent them replicating properly. Cyclophosphamide tends to affect B cells more than T cells, and there is some evidence that it also acts on Ig receptor renewal. It is effective in autoimmune diseases where antibody is a major factor (rheumatoid arthritis, SLE), but the common side-effect of sterility limits its use to older patients.

Methotrexate, fluorodeoxyuridine and *cytosine arabinoside* are other examples of drugs inhibiting DNA synthesis by interfering with various pathways, which have been considered as possible immunosuppressives.

Asparaginase, a bacterial enzyme, starves dividing lymphocytes (and tumour cells) of asparagine, bone marrow, etc. being spared.

Cyclosporin and *FK506* are important immunosuppressive agents obtained from fungi and bacteria, respectively. They bind to intracellular molecules called immunophilins, and in doing so block activation of the T-cell-specific transcription factor NF-AT, and hence the production of cytokines such as IL-2. Both have proved remarkably effective in bone marrow transplantation and have become the drugs of choice for most transplants, although long-term use is associated with a risk of kidney damage. Cyclosporin has the added advantage of killing a number of microorganisms that might otherwise infect the immunosuppressed host.

Plasma exchange (plasmapheresis), in which blood is removed and the cells separated from the plasma, and returned in dextran or some other plasma substitute, has been successful in acute crises of myasthenia gravis and Goodpasture's syndrome by reducing (usually only transiently) the level of circulating antibody or complexes. It is also life-saving in severe haemolytic disease of the newborn.

Corticosteroids (e.g. cortisone, prednisone) are, together with cyclosporin, the mainstay of organ transplant immunosuppression, and are also valuable in almost all hypersensitivity and autoimmune diseases. They can act on T cells, but their main effect is probably on polymorph and macrophage activity. Sodium retention (→ hypertension) and calcium loss (→ osteoporosis) are the major undesirable side effects.

Aspirin, indometacin, disodium cromoglicate (DSCG) and a variety of other anti-inflammatory drugs are useful in autoimmune diseases with an inflammatory component (for other ways to control type I hypersensitivity see Fig. 35).

Antibodies to inflammatory cytokines, especially TNF and IL-1 have proved powerful weapons in the treatment of chronic inflammatory diseases such as rheumatoid arthritis, Crohn's disease, psoriasis and gout. An alternative to antibodies is to use soluble forms of the cytokine receptors to 'mop up' free cytokine in the blood.

Specific immunosuppression

Antibody against **target antigens**, which is especially effective in preventing rejection of tumours, probably works by blocking class II determinants, which may also be how blood transfusion improves kidney graft survival (see Fig. 39). Anti-Rh (D) antibodies will prevent sensitization of Rh-negative mothers by removing the Rh-positive cells (see Fig. 36).

Antibody against the CD4 molecule on T cells, when administered at the same time as antigen, seems to induce a state of long-lasting antigen-specific tolerance, at least in animal models. A similar approach is being tried for prevention of transplant rejection in humans.

Antigen administered over a prolonged period in very low doses can induce antigen-specific tolerance. This approach, known as desensitization, has long been used for the suppression of allergies. However, because of the rare but dangerous risk of inducing anaphylaxis, it is seldom used in the UK. Antigen administered via the oral (and perhaps also nasal) route induces strong antigen-specific suppression in animals. A similar approach is being used in the treatment of autoimmune diseases; in one such trial patients with multiple sclerosis, in which autoimmune T cells attack the CNS, were fed extracts of animal myelin. Although some small therapeutic effects were observed, further testing has been disappointing.

Clonal elimination, or 'classic tolerance' (see Fig. 22), can be induced *in vitro* by coupling cytotoxic drugs or radioisotopes to antigen, which is then concentrated on the surface of those cells specifically binding it; some success has also been obtained *in vivo* with this 'retiarian therapy' (named after Roman warriors who caught their victims with a net and then killed them with a spear). It is quite possible that the suppression caused by antiproliferative drugs (e.g. cyclophosphamide, ciclosporin) in the presence of antigen, contains an element of specific clonal elimination.

Regulatory T cells Several research groups are also exploring the possibility of expanding the T^{REG} population, and hence inhibiting the specific immune response. However, one needs to proceed with caution. A recent trial on six volunteers at a London hospital ended in disaster, as an antibody that was supposed to stimulate expansion of T^{REG} cells in fact set off a 'cytokine storm' akin to a toxic shock reaction, resulting in severe damage to several of the volunteers.

41 Immunostimulation and vaccination

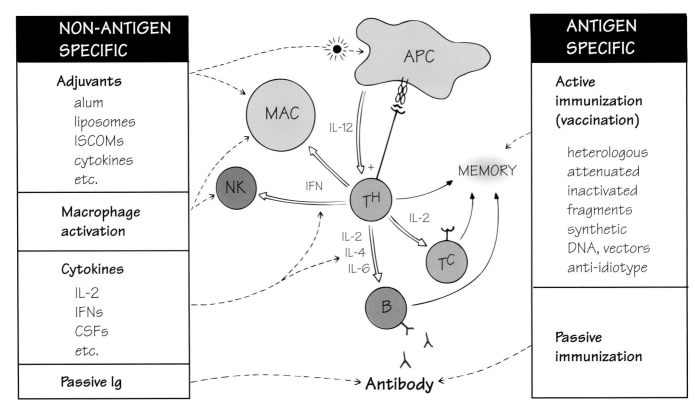

In most animals the combination of innate resistance and stimulation of adaptive responses by antigen is adequate to cope with common infections (otherwise the species would not survive!). However, the immune system does have its shortcomings, and some of these can be overcome by artificial means. Indeed, the introduction of vaccines has probably saved more lives than any other medical intervention to date. But there are still no effective vaccines against many of the world's most common infectious diseases, including HIV, tuberculosis and malaria.

Most effective vaccines need to stimulate both innate and adaptive immunity. Adaptive immune responses suffer from their initial slowness, so that high levels of antibody may arrive too late to prevent death or disability (e.g. tetanus, polio) even though surviving patients are resistant to reinfection. **Specific immunization** overcomes this problem by ensuring there is a high level of immunity **before** exposure. This may be **active** (top right), in which antigen is used to safely generate immunological memory, aided in some cases by the boosting power of special

non-specific stimulants or **adjuvants** (top left), or **passive**, in which preformed antibody is injected, with more rapid but short-lived effect.

Immunotherapy, as distinct from vaccination, refers to stimulating immune responses to cure, rather than prevent, disease. In general, conventional vaccines are ineffective when administered after exposure, although there are exceptions (rabies, chickenpox vaccination for prevention of shingles).

Finally, when some component of the immune system is deficient (see Fig. 33), efforts can be made to correct this by **replacement** of hormones, enzymes, cytokines, cells or organs.

Despite 200 years of cumulative success, there is a growing irrational fear of vaccination in the industrialized world and a corresponding rise in cases of dangerous illnesses such as measles and polio. Continued efforts at educating the public are required to ensure society benefits fully from the benefits of universal vaccination.

Target disease	Type of vaccine	Age of administration	Adjuvant
Diphtheria, tetanus, pertussis, Hib, polio	'5 in 1'	3–24 months	Alum
Measles, mumps, rubella (MMR)	Live attenuated	18–24 months (single)	None
Tuberculosis (BCG)	Live heterologous attenuated	Neonatal or in teenagers	None
Polio	Killed (Salk)	3–24 months	Alum
Haemophilus influenzae (Hib) (meningitis)	Polysaccharide conjugate	3–24 months	Alum
Meningococcus A/C	Polysaccharide/polysaccharide conjugate	3–24 months and 18–22 years	Alum
Hepatitis A and B	Subunit (recombinant)	High-risk groups only	Alum
Human papillomavirus	Subunit (recombinant)	Teenage girls	Alum and monophosphoryl lipid A

Adjuvants are materials that increase the response to an antigen given at the same time. One way in which many adjuvants work is by creating a slow-release depot of antigen, thus prolonging the time for which the immune system remains in contact with antigen. In addition, they contain substances that activate macrophages and dendritic cells and via this pathway also increase antigen presentation (see Fig. 18). The most powerful adjuvants (e.g. Freund's complete, which contains extracts of *Mycobacterium tuberculosis*) are too tissue-destructive for human use. Most human vaccines use a mixture of insoluble aluminium salts (alum) as adjuvant, but considerable efforts are being made to find more effective alternatives such as saponin.

Replacement therapy In some cases of severe combined immunodeficiency, bone marrow grafting has restored function; where adenosine deaminase (ADA) is deficient, this enzyme may also be restored by blood transfusion or, more recently, by gene therapy.

Cytokines Interferons, interleukins and other cytokines have potential for increasing the activity of their target cells, but their use in the clinic has been limited. IFNα has proved useful in certain viral diseases (e.g. hepatitis B and C), while G-CSF is used to boost granulocyte numbers after radiation or chemotherapy. However, the side effects of administering large amounts of cytokines systemically often limit their usefulness. More targeted cytokine release, e.g. by gene therapy, may prove more effective.

Passive immunization

Antibody In patients already exposed to disease, passively transferred antibody antiserum may be life-saving; examples are rabies, tetanus, hepatitis B and snake bite. Originally, antisera were raised in horses, but the danger of serum sickness (see Fig. 36) makes 'humanized' monoclonal antibodies (see Fig. 15) preferable wherever possible. Monoclonal antibodies against 'self' molecules have also proved remarkably effective in controlling some tumours (see Fig. 42). **T cells** are more difficult to administer, because they need to be obtained from the same individual to prevent rejection. However, T cells against cytomegalovirus, which are isolated from blood, stimulated with virus and cytokines, and then readministered to the patient, have proved useful in controlling this infection in immunosuppressed individuals (e.g. after transplantation).

Active immunization ('vaccination')

The term 'vaccine' was introduced by Pasteur to commemorate Jenner's classic work with cowpox (vaccinia), but was extended by him to all agents used to induce specific immunity and mitigate the effects of subsequent infection. Vaccines are given as early as practical, taking into account the fact that the immune system is not fully developed in the first months of life, and that antibody passively acquired from the mother via the placenta and/or milk will specifically prevent the baby making its own response. In general, this means a first injection at about 6 months, but where antibody is not of major importance (e.g. BCG) vaccines can be given effectively within 2 weeks of birth.

Living heterologous vaccines work by producing a milder but cross-protecting disease; one example is vaccinia, which has effectively allowed the elimination of smallpox. Another is BCG (attenuated bovine tuberculosis), which provides partial protection against tuberculosis especially when given to infants. However, with the rapid rise in tuberculosis worldwide, improved vaccines are urgently needed.

Living attenuated viruses (measles, mumps, yellow fever, rubella) produce subclinical disease and usually excellent protection. However, care is needed in immunodeficient patients. The measles, mumps and rubella vaccines are usually administered together (MMR). Public confidence in this vaccine was severely damaged by flawed research claiming a link between the vaccine and autism.

Inactivated vaccines are used where attenuation is not feasible; they include formalin-killed viruses such as rabies and influenza. The killed polio vaccine (Salk) has replaced the live (Sabin) vaccine in most countries.

Toxoids are bacterial toxins (e.g. diphtheria, tetanus) inactivated with formalin but still antigenic. These relatively simple vaccines have provided some of the most effective and reliable vaccines available to this day.

Capsular polysaccharides induce some (primarily IgM) antibody against meningococcal, pneumococcal and *Haemophilus* spp. infection. However, the level and persistence of protective antibody can be greatly enhanced by coupling the polysaccharide to protein antigens, which stimulate a strong 'helper' response. Tetanus or diphtheria toxoid is frequently used for this purpose. These 'conjugate' vaccines have proved of particular value in the fight against bacterial meningitis.

Subunit vaccines include the first of the 'second-generation' vaccines, in which the purified antigens are produced by recombinant DNA technology. The first examples of subunit vaccines were hepatitis A and B surface antigens and they provide a high (>90%) level of protection. A recombinant surface antigen vaccine against the sexually transmitted human papillomavirus was introduced in 2007 and prevents both viral infection and the subsequent development of cancer of the cervix, which is caused by this virus.

DNA, vectors An interesting idea is to insert genes from one microbe into another less virulent one such as vaccinia, attenuated *Salmonella* or even HIV-based 'viruses' which have been altered so as to prevent them replicating. These 'recombinant' organisms often stimulate strong immunity to the inserted antigens. If the vector has a large enough genome (e.g. BCG), multiple antigens could be introduced into a single vector, cutting down the need for repeated doses. A recent trial of such a 'recombinant' vaccine gave the first suggestion of protection against HIV infection. Some of the properties of the vaccines in common use are summarized in the table opposite (representing 2012 UK guidelines).

LIVERPOOL JOHN MOORES UNIVERSITY
LEARNING SERVICES

42 Cancer immunology

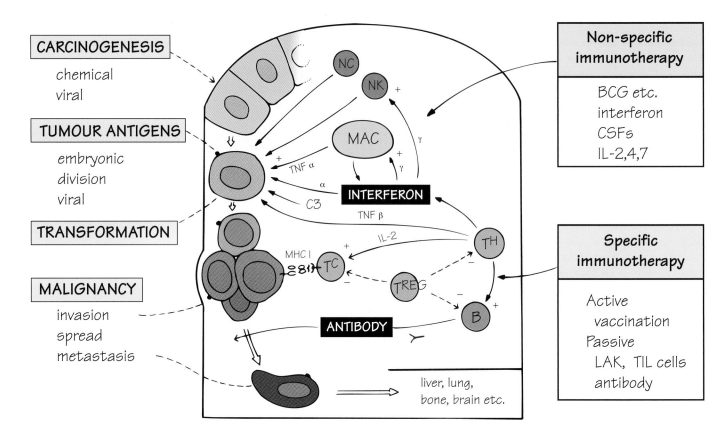

It has long been suspected that the immune system may be able to recognize tumours and destroy them, as it does an allogeneic transplant or a parasite. There is now good evidence for the old hypothesis that naturally occurring tumours are eliminated or contained by the immune system ('immune surveillance'). This hypothesis predicts that the frequency or progression of tumours increases in immunosuppressed individuals, a prediction that was initially borne out by studies on virally induced tumours, but has recently been extended to other more common types. Immunologists have therefore hoped that by appropriate stimulation of stronger innate or specific immunity (vaccination) the immune system could contribute to the eradication of cancer. In the last few years the enormous effort devoted to this problem has begun to be translated into some clinical successes and the mood is one of cautious optimism.

Many mechanisms can contribute to tumour control, including those of both innate (e.g. NK cells, macrophages, cytokines) and adaptive immunity. Attention has been focused on the identification of tumour-specific B- and T-cell antigens, although it now seems likely that tumour-associated antigens (TAAs), normal proteins found more frequently or at higher levels on tumour cells than on normal tissues, are equally important. Older research concentrated on the study of experimentally induced tumours in animals, but probably these very fast-growing and aggressive tumours are much easier for the immune system to recognize than the more typical human tumours that usually develop gradually over years or even decades. Instead, attempts are being made to identify the naturally occurring immune responses to tumours in patients with cancer.

Nevertheless, tumours continue to pose formidable challenges to the immunologist. In its relationship to the host, a tumour cell (yellow, brown and black in figure) is rather like a successful parasite, but with special additional features. Parasite-like mechanisms that help prevent elimination include **weak antigenicity** and extensive cross-reaction with self; **immunosuppression and tolerance induction**; release of **soluble antigens**; antigen–antibody **complexes**; and **antigenic variation**.

In mice, chemicals such as methylcholanthrene and benzopyrenes tend to induce tumours, each with unique 'idiotypic' antigens, whereas most of the common human cancers result from a slow and gradual accumulation of mutations in the genes of proteins that regulate the cell cycle. Such mutations can result in over-activation of a protein promoting cell growth (encoded by cellular *oncogenes*) or inactivation of a protein that normally slows down cell growth (encoded by *tumour-suppressor genes*). Some of these mutations are inherited, while others may result from exposure to chemicals in the environment. Normally, it requires several mutagenic events, which can occur over many decades, before a tumour develops. The mutated forms of these proteins may act as possible specific antigens for the adaptive immune system, especially the cytotoxic T cell.

Non-specific immunotherapy

BCG (an attenuated tubercle bacillus) has been tried against melanoma, sarcoma, etc., especially combined with other treatments. Its major immunological effect seems to be macrophage activation, but it may also affect NK cells. A tremendous range of bacterial and other immunostimulating agents has been tested for antitumour activity (see Fig. 41), but so far with very limited success.

Cytokines The dramatic effects of 'Coley's toxin' (a bacterial extract) 100 years ago may have been due to the vigorous induction of cytokines. Following the success of TNF in animals, numerous individual cytokines have also been tried on cancer patients. However, it is now becoming clear that inflammation, and excessive TNF-α production, can actually promote tumour growth, partly by increasing the blood supply to the tumour (angiogenesis). At present only IFNγ and IL-2 are in clinical use against some cancers, although a more targeted delivery to the site of the tumour (e.g. by gene therapy) may extend this approach.

MAC, NK Macrophages and natural killer cells (see Figs 8 and 15), especially when activated, can prevent growth of some tumours *in vitro* ('cytostasis') or actually kill them ('cytolysis'). NK cells are also cytotoxic, and are activated by cells that have lost expression of MHC molecules, a common phenotype of many tumours. IFNγ is important in activating macrophages and NK cells. Some tumour cells can apparently activate **complement** via the alternative pathway. However, note that there are potential dangers of activating macrophages and inflammation as discussed in the paragraph above.

Lymphocytes Tumours often contain large numbers of tumour-infiltrating lymphocytes (TILs), and the number and type of these cells can sometimes predict the rate of tumour progression. TILs are believed to be enriched for lymphocytes specifically recognizing the tumour cells, and such cells extracted from the tumour itself, expanded and then reinjected, have in some cases been successful in causing tumour rejection. Lymphocytes from the blood of tumour patients, activated non-specifically *in vitro* by IL-2 to kill (LAK cells) have also shown some promise.

Specific immunotherapy

Tumour antigens In the case of tumours induced by viruses, the **viral** antigens themselves are the target of the host immune response (see below). In non-viral tumours, the identification of TAAs has been much more difficult. In rare cases, **embryonic** antigens absent from normal adult cells may be re-expressed when they become malignant. Carcinoembryonic antigen (CEA) in the colon and α-fetoprotein in the liver are examples of diagnostic value. Other antigens found on the surface of some tumours are glycosylation variants of normal cell proteins (e.g. MUC-1 on epithelial tumours). However, it seems that the majority of antigens recognized by the host's cellular immune response are normal self proteins, which are expressed at higher concentrations than normal in the tumour cells (sometimes because they are required for cell division). Unfortunately, it seems as though tumours are very heterogeneous and antigens common to a large number of tumours have been difficult to identify.

Viruses were once thought to be responsible for many human tumors, but most common cancers are now thought not to be virally induced. However, five important forms of cancer are firmly linked to viruses (all DNA): Burkitt's lymphoma and nasopharyngeal carcinoma (EBV), Kaposi's sarcoma (KSHV), hepatocarcinoma (hepatitis B virus [HBV]) and cervical cancer (papillomavirus). RNA retroviruses may be responsible for some other cases. Interestingly, all these tumours increase in frequency in immunosuppressed individuals (Kaposi's sarcoma, for example, is commonly found in AIDS patients; see Fig. 28). Marek's disease, a tumour of chickens, was the first example of the introduction of a successful tumour vaccine. HBV vaccination lowers the risk of hepatocellular carcinoma by preventing viral infection, and a vaccine against papillomavirus prevents most cases of cervical cancer

Antibody There is little evidence that antibody normally provides any host immunity to tumours. Nevertheless, **passive immunization** using antibodies against two TAAs, CD20 on B-cell lymphomas and Her2/neu on epithelial cells, has been the first major success of tumour immunology, and these have entered the standard repertoire of drugs used by oncologists for treating these diseases. Much effort is underway to extend these successes to other tumours, and several other antibodies are in advanced stages of clinical trial. Another approach is to enhance the effectiveness of antibodies by coupling them to potent cytotoxic drugs ('magic bullet'). This aims to build up very high levels of anti-cancer drug in the immediate vicinity of the tumour, thus minimizing the general toxicity of the drug, which limits the concentrations that can normally be used for chemotherapy.

Cell-mediated immunity Cytotoxic CD8 T cells capable of lysing tumour cells *in vitro* have been isolated from both mice and humans (especially from individuals with melanoma). In mice such cytotoxic T cells can eliminate a tumour *in vivo*. Many tumours evade this by reducing their expression of MHC class I antigens. T^{H1} cells are also probably very important, because they can activate macrophages and NK cells via the release of IFNγ and are also essential for good CD8 T-cell memory. However, weak T-cell reactions may actually stimulate tumour growth and metastasis. Recent promising clinical **vaccination** trials using melanoma antigens have given a strong further impetus to this work, and there is also the possibility that T cells could be 'redirected' against a target tumor antigen by gene therapy of specific T-cell receptors (see Fig. 12).

Dendritic cells (see Fig. 4) are the most potent activators of cell-mediated immunity and it is therefore not surprising that many approaches have attempted to harness these cells for immunotherapy. One approach is to isolate dendritic cells from a patient, load them with tumour antigens and then reintroduce them into the body. Although these patient-specific **adoptive immunotherapy** procedures are difficult and expensive to implement, a dendritic cell-based immunotherapy for prostate cancer has recently been licenced in the USA, and further treatments of this type are likely to follow.

Breaking tolerance The immune response to most tumours is probably limited by the strong regulatory mechanisms that operate to prevent autoimmunity and maintain tolerance (see Fig. 22). Many strategies aimed at interfering with these mechanisms, and hence obtaining more effective immune responses are being explored. These include blocking molecules on the T-cell surface such as CTLA4 which transmit negative signals, depleting T^{REG} cells and using gene therapy to produce large populations of T cells that carry specific receptors for tumour antigens. New biological drugs based on these strategies are now entering the clinic, and there is great excitement about their potential. Note that treatments may involve some unavoidable side effects in the form of autoimmunity (see Fig. 38).

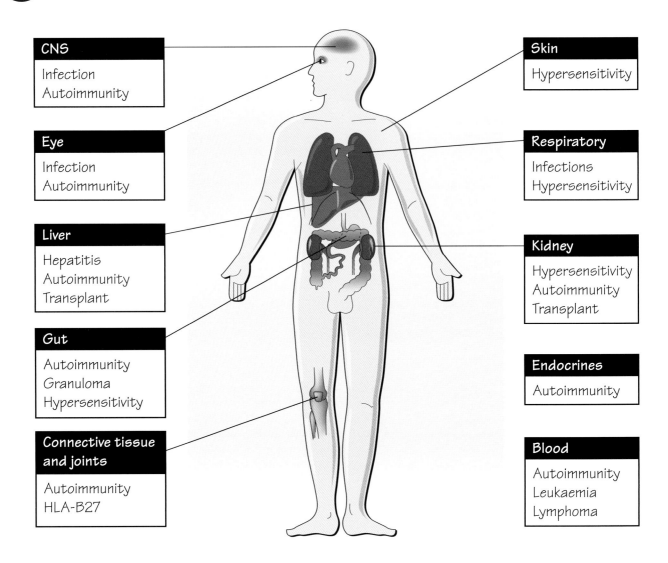

CNS
Infection
Autoimmunity

Eye
Infection
Autoimmunity

Liver
Hepatitis
Autoimmunity
Transplant

Gut
Autoimmunity
Granuloma
Hypersensitivity

Connective tissue and joints
Autoimmunity
HLA-B27

Skin
Hypersensitivity

Respiratory
Infections
Hypersensitivity

Kidney
Hypersensitivity
Autoimmunity
Transplant

Endocrines
Autoimmunity

Blood
Autoimmunity
Leukaemia
Lymphoma

Clinical immunology is a specialty in its own right and there are many excellent textbooks devoted to it. Here we can only summarize the most common conditions encountered by the clinical immunologist, arranged by **organs** and/or **systems** rather than, as elsewhere in this book, by **mechanism**. Obviously there are frequent overlaps with other disciplines, which is why the clinical immunologist is expected to be familiar with all branches of pathology and medicine. For example, a case of myeloma could present to the accident and emergency department (A&E) with a fracture or be referred to the rheumatology department because of bone pain, to urology because of renal failure, to haematology because of anaemia, to immunology because of immunodeficiency, or even to the neurology or eye clinic. Abnormalities may be picked up by the radiologist, by the haematologist in a marrow biopsy, or simply from serum electrophoresis or a urine test. In the same way any patient with liver, kidney, lung, joint or skin disease, or with an unusual infection, should be looked at with the immunological possibilities in mind. The figure can be used as a checklist; brief details are provided on the opposite page. Remember that immune status is critical when considering vaccination, transplantation and in monitoring the course of AIDS.

CNS Blood–brain barrier keeps out most infections.
- Meningitis: usually bacterial; encephalitis more often viral (NB prions: Creutzfeldt–Jakob disease [CJD]).
- Multiple sclerosis: plaques of demyelination in brain, with Ig in cerebrospinal fluid (CSF); progressive with remissions, IFNβ delays progression.
- Guillain–Barré syndrome: demyelination in peripheral nerve post infection; normally complete recovery.
- Myasthenia gravis: autoimmune destruction of acetylcholine receptors at nerve–muscle junction; muscle fatigue; maternal antibody can affect neonate; plasmapheresis to remove antibody.

Eye The eye, open to the air, is protected from infection by tears, lysozyme and IgA.
- Common infections: adenovirus, *Streptococcus pneumoniae* (conjunctiva), trachoma (eyelid), CMV, *Toxoplasma* spp. (retina), congenital rubella (lens).
- Uveitis: common in rheumatic and other systemic autoimmune diseases.
- Sympathetic ophthalmia after unilateral damage.
- Corneal grafts: 65% non-rejection.

Liver
- Hepatitis B and C: damage to liver cells by chronic cytotoxic T-cell activation, not by virus; 10% (B) and 50% (C) become carriers. Persistent 'chronic active' disease, may lead to cirrhosis, carcinoma. Congenital adrenal hyperplasia (CAH) may also be autoimmune, Wilson's disease (copper), haemochromatosis (iron). Hepatitis A and B vaccines available.
- Primary biliary cirrhosis: autoimmune, with antimitochondrial antibodies; probably bacterial cross-reaction.
- Possibility of transplant for liver failure.

Gut
- Sjögren's syndrome: salivary gland autoimmunity; dry mouth.
- Pernicious anaemia: autoimmune gastritis plus antibody to intrinsic factor; vitamin B_{12} not absorbed.
- Coeliac disease: α-gliadin hypersensitivity leading to jejunal malabsorption. Controlled by gluten-free diet.
- Crohn's disease: constricting granulomas in small intestine. May result from granulocyte functional deficit.
- Ulcerative colitis: ulcers may bleed. Both ulcerative colitis and Crohn's disease show lymphocytic infiltration.

Connective tissue and joints
- Rheumatoid arthritis: IgM antibodies to IgG (rheumatoid factor [RF]) in 70%, suggestive but not diagnostic. No infectious cause identified. May be changes in lung, skin, blood vessels, etc. T cells, plasma cells, macrophages, cytokines in joints. Blocking TNF effective.
- Seronegative arthritis (i.e. no RF): includes ankylosing spondylitis (90 times greater risk if HLA-B27) and Reiter's disease (post bowel or genitourinary infection – 'reactive' arthritis).
- Systemic lupus erythematosus: multiorgan pathology (lung, kidney, skin rash, brain); antibodies to nuclei (ANA), dsDNA, 25% have RF. High circulating interferon levels. Some cases due to drugs.
- Systemic sclerosis: multiorgan, may have RF, ANA, CREST syndrome (**c**alcinosis, **R**aynaud's, **o**esophageal dysmotility, **s**clerodactyly, **t**elangiectasia).
- Polymyositis: muscle and joint lesions.
- Dermatomyositis: muscle, joints, skin.

Skin
- Hypersensitivities common, e.g. type I, urticaria (IgE, mast cells); type II, bullous diseases (autoantibody); type III, vasculitis (immune complexes); type IV, contact dermatitis (T cells, cytokines).
- Atopic eczema: multiple allergies.
- Skin rashes may be cytopathic (smallpox), toxic (*Streptococcus* spp.), immunological (measles).

Respiratory system Open to pathogens; alveoli protected by: (i) mucociliary escalator; (ii) alveolar macrophages; (iii) alveolar surfactants; and (iv) IgA.
- Upper respiratory infection: mainly viral, plus streptococci, *Haemophilus* spp.; spread to sinuses, ear.
- Pneumonia: many viruses, bacteria; especially common in immunodeficiency (antibody defect – capsulated bacteria; T-cell defect – tuberculosis).
- Sarcoidosis: lung granulomas, cause unknown.
- Hypersensitivities common, e.g. type I, allergic asthma; type II, Goodpasture's syndrome (autoantibody, also glomerulus); type III, extrinsic allergic alveolitis (e.g. farmer's lung); type IV, granulomas (e.g. tuberculosis). Lung fibrosis also from silica, asbestos, etc.
- Adult respiratory distress syndrome (ARDS) in acute shock; may involve inflammatory cytokines (TNF, etc.).

Kidney Glomerulonephritis is usually immunological.
- Immune complex mediated, e.g. post-streptococcal infection, anti-DNA in SLE, also unidentified IgA complexes.
- Autoimmune: antibody to basement membrane in Goodpasture's syndrome. Also antibody to tubular basement membrane.
- Kidney involved in many vascular diseases.
- Transplantation the ideal treatment for renal failure; importance of HLA matching.

Endocrine organs Most endocrine disease due to autoimmunity; more common in women than men. Considerable disease overlap in individuals and relatives; some influence of HLA type. Treatment relatively simple with hormone replacement.
- Thyroid: most thyrotoxicosis due to autoantibody stimulating TSH receptor. Other autoantibodies may block receptor. Hashimoto's disease: autoimmune destruction of some or all of thyroid. Many autoantibodies found but pathogenicity uncertain.
- Pancreas: type 1 (insulin-dependent) diabetes due to T-cell destruction of islet β cells; also autoantibodies to islets and insulin.
- Adrenal cortex: autoimmunity now the commonest cause of Addison's disease; mainly T-cell-mediated destruction of gland.
- Testis: damage to testis (e.g. by trauma, mumps virus) can release sperm antigens, leading to autoimmunity and (rarely) infertility.

Blood
- Anaemia, neutropenia and thrombocytopenia may be autoimmune (for pernicious anaemia see above). In haemolytic anaemia, 'warm' antibodies mainly IgG anti-Rhesus; 'cold' IgM anti-I (paroxysmal cold haemoglobinuria). (Note: haemolysis may also be due to mismatched transfusion!)
- In treated haemophilia there may be antibodies to factor VIII.
- Myeloma: tumour of plasma cells; monoclonal paraproteins, IgG or IgA.
- Lymphocytic leukaemias: monoclonal tumours of lymphocyte series, mostly B, some T (acute: immature; chronic: mature).
- Lymphomas: solid lymphoid tumours.
  - (a) Hodgkin's: lymph node, spleen; cell of origin probably B.
  - (b) Non-Hodgkin's: very heterogeneous, B, T, NK or mixture.
  - (c) Burkitt's: B-cell tumour, associated with EBV infection, malaria, immunodeficiency.
  - (d) T cell (rare): may be due to HTLV-I.

44 Investigating immunity

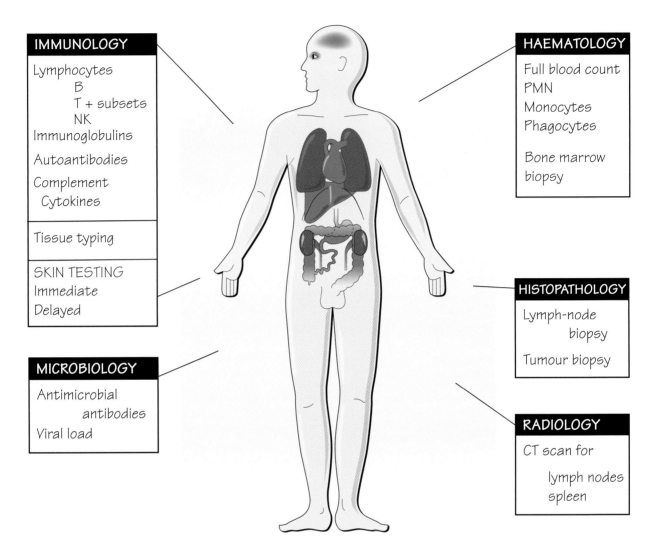

IMMUNOLOGY

Lymphocytes
 B
 T + subsets
 NK
Immunoglobulins

Autoantibodies

Complement
 Cytokines

Tissue typing

SKIN TESTING
Immediate
Delayed

MICROBIOLOGY

Antimicrobial
 antibodies
Viral load

HAEMATOLOGY

Full blood count
PMN
Monocytes
Phagocytes

Bone marrow
biopsy

HISTOPATHOLOGY

Lymph-node
 biopsy

Tumour biopsy

RADIOLOGY

CT scan for
 lymph nodes
 spleen

As most of the cells and molecules of the immune system spend some or all of their time in the blood, sampling them is usually straightforward, and the standard tests illustrated here account for a substantial part of the routine work of the immunology and haematology laboratories, and often of microbiology and biochemistry too. The assays are mainly automated and a report will usually give the normal values and indicate which results are abnormal. Nevertheless, because of the considerable differences between individuals, and in the same individual with time, interpretation is not always obvious, even to those well versed in other aspects of medicine. The interpretation of tests for autoimmunity is particularly tricky.

Assays of both immunological molecules (e.g. antibody) and cells mainly make use of standard reagents, which are themselves frequently monoclonal antibodies, designed to react with only one molecular feature or cell-surface marker. The use of antibodies, whether monoclonal or not, to detect antigens of any kind is referred to as **immunoassay** (see Fig. 45). For detection, antibodies may be labelled with a radio-isotope (radioimmunoassay), an enzyme (ELISA) or a fluorescent molecule (immunofluorescence).

Occasionally, something more elaborate may be requested, e.g. a skin test for hypersensitivity, a bone marrow or other organ biopsy, blood or tissue typing before a transfusion or an organ graft, or the analysis of a leukaemia. Immunological tests are also used in epidemiology, e.g. to assess the extent of epidemics or the success of vaccines, and for the diagnosis of infections where the pathogen itself is not easily detected. In general, IgM antibodies denote recent, and IgG past, exposure.

Both the immune system and pathogens are increasingly studied through **genes** (see Fig. 47). Many diagnostic tests now rely on the PCR (see Fig. 45) to detect specific pathogens. High throughput techniques make it feasible to measure and analyse thousands of different proteins, genes and metabolites in tiny samples of tissue or blood: in the medicine of the future, these technologies will be used increasingly for diagnosis, and the development of ever more individualized medical treatments.

Investigating immunodeficiency (see also Fig. 33)

Antibody deficiencies Total immunoglobulins and individual classes (e.g. IgG, IgA) can be measured by nephelometry or turbidimetry, ELISA, etc. A complete lack of immunoglobulins can be detected by absence of the γ-globulin arc in gel electrophoresis. Levels of antibody against particular antigens (e.g. a candidate virus) are measured by ELISA.

Lymphocyte deficiencies Total lymphocytes are counted by standard haematological methods. B and T lymphocytes are analysed by staining with fluorescent monoclonal antibodies against characteristic surface markers (e.g. CD3, CD4, CD8 for T cells and subsets, CD20 for B cells) combined with flow cytometry (see Fig. 45). Antigen-specific T-cell responses can be investigated in the clinic using a delayed hypersensitivity skin test, a common example being the Mantoux or Heaf test for prior exposure to tuberculosis, read 48–72 hours after injection. An alternative is to measure the proportion of blood producing production of a cytokine (such as IFNγ) in response to an antigen challenge.

Complement deficiencies Individual components, mainly C3, C4 and C1, are measured as for antibody. The functions of the lytic pathway can be assessed by haemolysis of antibody-coated red cells. Complement consumption ('fixation') by immune complexes is still sometimes used in estimating antibody levels in infections.

Phagocyte deficiencies Neutrophils and monocytes are counted as a routine part of a full blood count. Neutrophil function can be studied using the nitroblue tetrazolium (NBT) test, which measures the 'respiratory burst', or by the intracellular killing of selected bacteria.

Investigating allergy (see also Fig. 35)

Serum IgE Total and antigen-specific IgE are measured by a solid-phase fluorescent ELISA 'capture' assay.

Skin testing Immediate hypersensitivity, a reddened wheal 10–20 minutes after intradermal injection of the allergen, denotes the presence of specific IgE on mast cells in the skin. This is the most widely used initial test for allergies. For contact sensitivity, a patch test is used.

Investigating autoimmunity (see also Fig. 38)

Anti-Ig (rheumatoid factor) is detected by agglutination of Ig-coated red cells or latex particles, or by nephelometry/turbidimetry. Antibodies to cellular antigens are detected by immunofluoresence on sections of various tissues, which often shows a pattern characteristic of particular autoantibodies, e.g. antinuclear, antimitochondrial, antibasement membrane. This can be refined by ELISA using specific antigens, e.g. double-stranded DNA.

Note that the association between particular autoantibodies and particular diseases, though often highly suggestive, is seldom 100% positive.

Tissue typing and transplantation (see also Fig. 39)

HLA (see Fig. 11) is extremely polymorphic, and matching the specific alleles carried by a donor and a recipient is a key determinant of success in many types of transplantation. This process is known as 'tissue typing' and is now performed routinely by characterizing the specific class I and II gene variants using PCR.

Detection of antibody Patients who have been transfused or have rejected a previous graft may already possess antibodies against HLA antigens. These can be detected by reacting them with a panel of donors, or a single potential donor if one has already been identified.

Blood transfusion Fortunately, red cells do not carry HLA antigens, and normally the only antigens for which matching is essential are A, B, O and RhD. Note that ABO matching is as critical for the survival of an organ graft as it is for a pint of blood.

Tumours of immunological cells

Leukaemias can usually be identified by flow cytometry using paired antibodies specific for surface markers (see Fig. 45). For example, chronic B-cell leukemias often carry both CD5 and CD20, while acute B-cell leukaemias carry CD10 and CD19.

Lymphomas can usually be typed in tissue sections using fluorescent or enzyme-linked antibodies.

Myeloma This tumour of plasma cells can be recognized by the presence of a prominent monoclonal 'spike' in serum electrophoresis, and class-specific antisera can be used to identify the heavy and light chain class. The diagnosis can be confirmed by bone marrow biopsy.

Table of common normal adult values (note: these may vary from lab to lab)	
Lymphocytes	28–39% of white blood cells; 1600–2400 per mm^3
	T 67–76 % of lymphocytes; 1100–1700 per mm^3
	B 11–16% of lymphocytes; 200–400 per mm^3
NK cells	10–19% of 'lymphocytes'; 200–400 per mm^3
Phagocytic cells	PMN: 1800–7700 per mm^3
	Monocytes: 200–800 per mm^3
Immunoglobulins (serum)	IgG 5.3–16.5 g/L
	IgM 0.5–2.0 g/L (newborn: 0.05–0.2 g/L)
	IgA 0.8–4.0 g/L (newborn: 0.01–0.08 g/L)
	IgE 0.05 mg/L

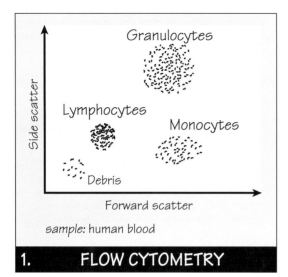

sample: human blood

1. **FLOW CYTOMETRY**

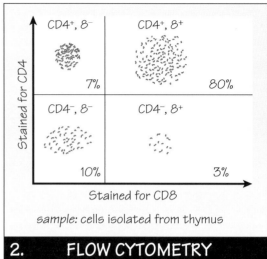

sample: cells isolated from thymus

2. **FLOW CYTOMETRY**

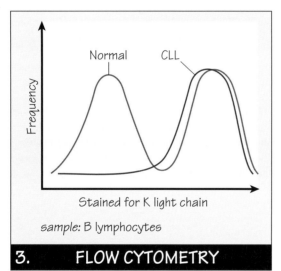

sample: B lymphocytes

3. **FLOW CYTOMETRY**

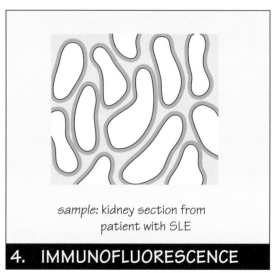

sample: kidney section from patient with SLE

4. **IMMUNOFLUORESCENCE**

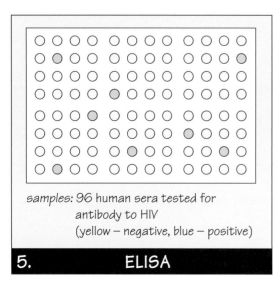

samples: 96 human sera tested for antibody to HIV
(yellow – negative, blue – positive)

5. **ELISA**

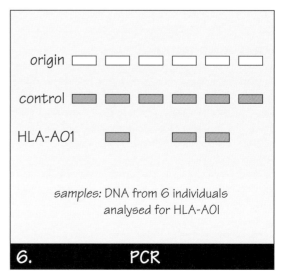

samples: DNA from 6 individuals analysed for HLA-AOl

6. **PCR**

The ability to measure accurately and sensitively different aspects of immunological function is an important part of both experimental and clinical immunology (see Chapter 44). Some of the most commonly used techniques in the immunological laboratory (immunological assays) are shown in the figure. Some techniques, such as the differential blood count, have hardly changed in over a hundred years. Others, such as flow cytometry and the PCR continue to evolve at a rapid rate as new technologies are developed. In all cases, clinical laboratories are making increased use of robotics and sophisticated computational analysis to automate all aspects of the process, to make it faster, cheaper and more reliable. The ability to integrate many different measurements (immunological, haematological, psychological, genetic, etc.) taken from each patient rapidly and reliably is also driving the development of 'personalized medicine', where doctors will be increasingly able to tailor each treatment precisely to match the needs of individual patients.

Flow cytometry (Fig. 45.1–45.3) is one of the most powerful techniques in the immunologist's repertoire. Cells are sucked into a fine jet of liquid so that they pass rapidly across a beam of one or, in more sophisticated machines, several lasers. Cells scatter the incoming beam of light by refraction and reflection. Light scattered through a small angle is called 'forward scatter' and is proportional to the size of the cells. Light scattered through a 90° angle is called 'side scatter' and depends on the granularity of the cell; e.g. a granulocyte has a much larger side scatter than a lymphocyte (see Fig. 45.1).

Cells can also be mixed with mixed with antibodies that bind to specific molecules on the cell's surface. Each antibody is linked to a molecule (fluorophore) with the property of absorbing light of one wavelength and re-emitting it at another. Many such molecules exist, some originally isolated from marine organisms. Light emitted by each cell is collected by a series of mirrors and then detected by one of several photomultipliers and stored on a computer. The precise composition of the mixture of cells can then be determined by analysis of their signals. In Fig. 45.2, cells from the thymus are shown as positive for CD4, CD8, both, or neither. The results can be displayed in the form of a dot plot (Fig. 45.1 and 45.2) in which each cell is represented as a dot, or as a histogram (Fig. 45.3). Results from histogram analyses can be superimposed as in Fig. 45.3, permitting easy comparisons between healthy and disease samples (e.g. blood cells from patients with leukaemia as shown in figure).

In a further refinement, cells binding different antibodies can be collected in separate tubes (fluorescence-activated cell sorting [FACS]), a powerful tool for isolating very pure cell populations from a mixture.

Immunofluorescence (Fig. 45.4), in addition to its role in flow cytometry, can also be applied to histological specimens, commonly to identify autoantibodies or immune complexes, or metastatic cancer cells invading healthy tissues. Figure 45.4 shows a kidney from a patient with systemic lupus erythematosus stained with a fluorescent antibody to IgG, which has bound to the immune complexes along the basement membrane.

ELISA (Fig. 45.5) The enzyme-linked immunoabsorbent assay is one of the most versatile immunological techniques. In direct ELISA, a target antigen, e.g. microbial proteins, or human DNA, is adsorbed on to a plastic surface – typically 96 or 396 small 'wells' – allowing many samples to be tested simultaneously. Diluted samples of serum to be tested are added, and any antibodies specific for the target antigen will become bound and immobilized to the plastic surface. Unbound serum components are then washed off and a 'second' antibody, e.g. to human Ig, which has been linked to an enzyme is added. An enzyme is chosen that converts a colourless substrate to a coloured product, which can then be measured in a spectrophotometer. Direct ELISA is often used to detect antibodies to microbes in infection (Fig. 45.5 shows the results of testing different human sera for the presence of antibodies to HIV) or to self antigens in autoimmune disease.

Sandwich ELISA In another variant, a specific antibody is first adsorbed to the plastic wells, then the serum or other sample to be tested, and finally the enzyme-linked second antibody, so as to form an antibody–antigen–antibody 'sandwich'. Complement components, cytokines, etc. can be conveniently assayed in this way. Much effort is being put into improved ELISA-like protocols that have increased sensitivity and can detect many components in a single sample (known as 'multiplexing'), reducing sample size, speed and cost.

PCR (Fig. 45.6) The PCR is the most recent addition to the immunology laboratory. The basic principle is to replicate any desired piece of DNA or RNA and make enough copies of it to be easily detected, sequenced and characterized. The simple and elegant technique consists of three steps. The target DNA (known as the template) is heated to 94°C so as to separate the two strands of double helix (**denaturation**), and mixed with two very short pieces of DNA (known as **primers**), which each have a sequence complementary to one end of the piece of DNA to be amplified. One primer is complementary to a specific sequence on one strand of DNA, while the second matches a sequence on the complementary strand in the opposite direction. The temperature is lowered so the primers bind to their complementary matching sequences on the template (**annealing**). The DNA is replicated (**extension**), using a special polymerase (often known as Taq), which was originally isolated from thermophilic bacteria living in deep oceanic hot springs, and which therefore works well at very high temperatures. The polymerase uses the primers as starting points to replicate a few hundred to a few thousand bases of the DNA. The cycle is then repeated, each time doubling the number of copies of the DNA sequence that lie between the two primers. The technique is so sensitive it can be used to detect a single copy of starting DNA. PCR has become the standard approach to HLA typing (see Figs 11 and 44). The technique can be modified so it gives a quantitative measurement of the amount of template in the starting material (qPCR), and is now used routinely to measure levels of virus or bacteria in samples of blood or other tissues.

46 Out of the past: evolution of immune mechanisms

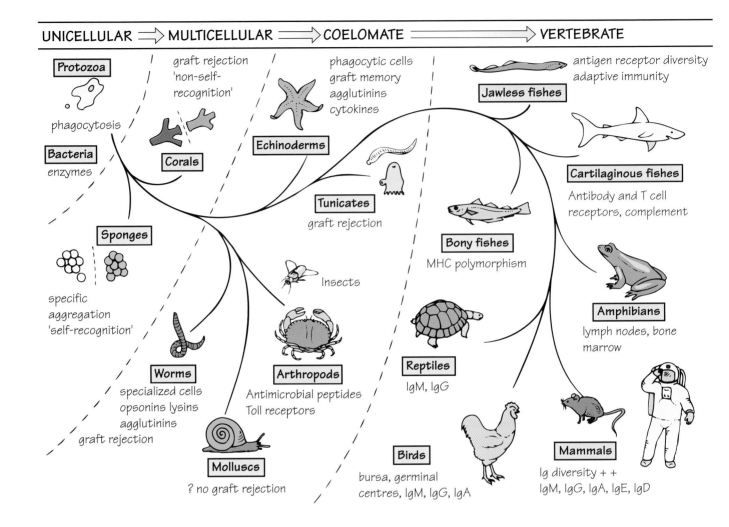

UNICELLULAR ⟹ MULTICELLULAR ⟹ COELOMATE ⟹ VERTEBRATE

Protozoa
phagocytosis

Bacteria
enzymes

graft rejection 'non-self-recognition'

Corals

phagocytic cells
graft memory
agglutinins
cytokines

Echinoderms

Jawless fishes
antigen receptor diversity
adaptive immunity

Cartilaginous fishes
Antibody and T cell receptors, complement

Tunicates
graft rejection

Sponges
specific aggregation 'self-recognition'

Insects

Bony fishes
MHC polymorphism

Amphibians
lymph nodes, bone marrow

Worms
specialized cells
opsonins lysins
agglutinins
graft rejection

Arthropods
Antimicrobial peptides
Toll receptors

Reptiles
IgM, IgG

Molluscs
? no graft rejection

Birds
bursa, germinal centres, IgM, IgG, IgA

Mammals
Ig diversity + +
IgM, IgG, IgA, IgE, IgD

From the humble amoeba searching for food (top left) to the mammal with its sophisticated humoral and cellular immune mechanisms (bottom right), all cellular organisms can discriminate between self and non-self, and have developed defence systems to prevent their cells and tissues being colonized by parasites.

This figure shows some of the important landmarks in the evolution of immunity. As most advances, once achieved, persist in subsequent species, they have for clarity been shown only where they are first thought to have appeared. It must be remembered that our knowledge of primitive animals is based largely on study of their modern descendants, all of whom evidently have immune systems adequate to their circumstances.

All multicellular organisms, including plants, have evolved a variety of recognition systems that respond to common molecular patterns found on the surface of microbes (e.g. lipopolysaccharides) by stimulating a variety of antimicrobial responses. This broadly corresponds to vertebrate innate immunity. In contrast, only vertebrates appear to have evolved adaptive immunity (characterized by specificity and memory), mediated by lymphocytes and three separate recognition systems (see Fig. 3): molecules expressed on B cells only (antibody), on T cells only (the T-cell receptor) and on a range of cells (the MHC), all of which look as if their genes evolved from a single primitive precursor (for further details see Fig. 10). Why only vertebrates have evolved adaptive immunity has never been totally explained, but there is a growing appreciation that the adaptive immune system brings with it very significant evolutionary costs. These include energy demands in maintaining the system (the human immune system has at least as many cells as the human nervous system), and also the potential danger that excess immunity will lead to tissue damage (as outlined in Figs 34–39). One of the consequences of the evolutionary quest to balance the pros and cons of the immune system is reflected in the extraordinary evolutionary diversity and genetic variability in many families of molecules involved in immune function (see Fig. 47).

Unicellular organisms

Bacteria We think of bacteria as parasites, but they themselves can be infected by specialized viruses called **bacteriophages** and have developed sophisticated systems to prevent this. It is thought that the restriction endonucleases, so indispensable to the modern genetic engineer, have as their real function the recognition and destruction of viral DNA without damage to that of the host bacterium. Successful bacteriophages have evolved resistance to this, a beautiful example of innate immunity and its limitations.

Protozoa Lacking chlorophyll, these little animals must eat. Little is known about how they recognize 'food', but their surface proteins are under quite complex genetic control.

Invertebrates

Research in this area is very active, partly because it has become clear that some invertebrates make very useful models for the study of vertebrate innate immunity, and partly because of the importance of some invertebrates in carrying human diseases (e.g. malaria transmission by mosquitoes).

Sponges and corals. Partly free-living, partly colonial, sponge *and coral* cells use species-specific glycoproteins to identify 'self' and prevent hybrid colony formation. If forced together, non-identical colonies undergo necrosis at the contact zone, with accelerated breakdown of a second graft.

Worms Because of its relative simplicity and ease of propagation, the nematode *Caenorhabditis elegans* has become one of the most thoroughly studied animals on earth. Protection against infection is achieved by behavioural responses (mediated by a **Toll receptor;** see Fig. 5), a thick outer coat or cuticle and production of a range of soluble antimicrobial peptides and proteins.

Molluscs and arthropods are curious in apparently not showing graft rejection. However, both cellular and humoral immunity are present. An important humoral system involves the enzyme prophenyl oxidase, which is involved in production of toxic oxygen radicals and melanin, both thought to play a part in defence against potential pathogens. A common cellular response is encapsulation, in which invading microorganisms are rapidly surrounded by blood cells and sealed off, thus preventing spread of infection. A key feature of the insect immune response (studied especially in the fruit fly *Drosophila melanogaster*) is the production of an amazing number of different antimicrobial peptides. Two major cellular signalling pathways are involved in switching on the production of these peptides, the Toll receptor pathway, which also plays an important part in mediating **innate immunity** in vertebrates, and the Imd pathway, which shares many features with the vertebrate **tumour necrosis factor** pathway.

Echinoderms The starfish is famous for Metchnikoff's classic demonstration of specialized phagocytic cells in 1882. Allografts (grafts from one individual to another) are rejected, with cellular infiltration, and there is a strong specific memory response.

Tunicates (e.g. *Amphioxus,* sea-squirts) These pre-vertebrates show several advanced features: self-renewing haemopoietic cells, lymphoid-like cells, and a single gene complex controlling the rejection of foreign grafts. Most of the major components of the complement pathway are also first found in this group of animals. Although none of the major components of adaptive immunity have been found in any invertebrate, other molecules of the 'immunoglobulin superfamily', e.g. adhesion molecules, are already present in invertebrates.

Vertebrates

Jawless fishes (cyclostomes, e.g. hagfish, lamprey) These descendents of the earliest vertebrates lack the immunoglobulin-based adaptive immune system. In a remarkable example of parallel evolution, they were recently shown to have two classes of lymphocytes, analogous to T and B cells, but to use a different type of variable lymphocyte receptor based on the leucine rich domain structure (see Fig. 5).

Cartilaginous fishes (e.g. sharks) The evolution of the jawed vertebrates marks the first appearance of classic antibody, T-cell antigen receptors and MHC, although details of isotype, isotype switching and somatic recombination differ from higher vertebrates. Many molecules of the classic complement pathway also make their appearance.

Bony fish Bony fish have most of the features of immunity familiar to us from a study of humans and mice. The zebra fish has become an attractive model species for the study of immunity and inflammation, because its transparent body structure allows high resolution imaging, and its small size facilitates the development of rapid screening assays for new immunomodulatory drugs. Interest in fish immunology has also been driven by economic considerations, as infectious diseases pose a major challenge for farmed fish such as salmon.

Amphibians During morphogenesis (e.g. tadpole → frog) specific tolerance develops towards the new antigens of the adult stage. Lymph nodes and gut-associated lymphoid tissue (GALT) and haemopoiesis in the bone marrow also appear for the first time.

Birds are unusual in producing their B lymphocytes exclusively in a special organ, the bursa of Fabricius, near the cloaca. The mechanisms for generating different antibody molecules also seem to be quite different, involving a process known as **gene conversion**. They have a large multilobular thymus but no conventional lymph nodes.

Reptiles have both T and B cells. As in birds, the major antibody class is IgY rather than IgG, although both IgM, IgD and possibly IgA may also exist.

Mammals are characterized more by diversity of Ig classes and subclasses, and MHC antigens, than by any further development of effector functions. There are some curious variations; e.g. rats have unusually strong innate immunity and some animals (whales, Syrian hamsters) show surprisingly little MHC polymorphism. However, humans and mice, fortunately (for the humans), are immunologically remarkably similar. Members of the cammelid family (e.g. camels and llamas) have antibodies made up of a single heavy chain and no light chain (see Fig. 14).

Plants

Plants, like animals, possess sophisticated mechanisms to protect themselves against microbial pathogens. These responses are triggered by plant receptors that recognize molecular components of bacteria, fungi or viruses. The responses include secretion of a variety of antimicrobial substances, some of which (e.g. nitric oxide) are shared with vertebrate immunity. RNA silencing, in which short stretches of double-stranded RNA can trigger sequence-specific mRNA degradation, and hence gene silencing, forms part of another elaborate antiviral immune system in plants.

Into the future: immunology in the age of genomics

47

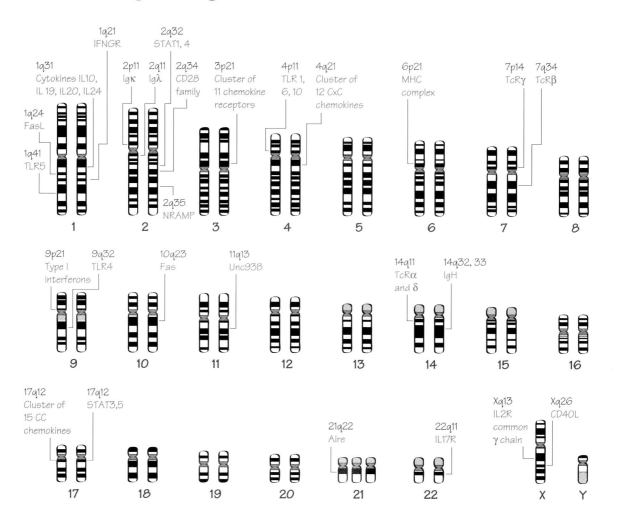

The completion of the first complete DNA sequence of the human genome in 2003 was a landmark in the history of science. Remarkably, despite containing over 3 billion base pairs, the genome is believed to code for only around 20000 genes, far fewer than most scientists had estimated. The function of much of the rest of the DNA remains unclear, although much of it is likely to be involved in regulating gene expression. An increasing number of genomes of other organisms (including of course the indispensable laboratory mouse) are already, or will be shortly be, available. Genome-wide comparisons between species are already providing fascinating new insights into the process of evolution. The next major phase of the genome project, to define the diversity of the DNA sequence within a species, is now under way. Current data suggest that the DNA sequences of any two humans differ from each other by an amazing 10000000 base pairs. The most common type of difference are called single nucleotide substitutions, or SNPs, (pronounced 'snips').

All this information has had a major impact on immunology, allowing rapid discovery of many new molecules involved in the interaction between the host and the pathogen. The figure shows the 22 human autosomes, plus the X and Y chromosome, stained with a DNA dye that gives a characteristic banding pattern known as the ideogram. Each band is given a number (e.g. 14q32 means band 32 on the long arm of chromosome 14, p refers to the short arm) which unambiguously identifies that region of the chromosome. The figure illustrates in green the ideogram positions of the genes that code for some of the most important molecules making up the human immune system, all of which are discussed elsewhere in this book. One striking discovery, illustrated in this figure, is the extent to which the immune system is made up of multigene families, which have presumably arisen by multiple duplication events. Many immune genes are also polymorphic. The extent of immune gene duplication and polymorphism (far greater than in most non-immune genes) is testament to the enormous selective pressure exerted by the microbial world during our past evolutionary history. Mutations in several genes have been associated with (often very rare) diseases affecting the immune system. The list is not exclusive, as new examples are rapidly being discovered. You can find information about any other gene you may be interested in by searching at the American National Centre for Biotechnology Information http://www.ncbi.nlm.nih.gov/projects/mapview/.

Knowledge of one's own genome and of its likely gene associations will offer exciting and extraordinary possibilities, but also disturbing ethical challenges, to both the medical profession and the individual.

T-cell receptors T lymphocytes recognize antigen using a two-chain receptor made up either of **γ/δ** or, much more commonly, **α/β** chains. These genes, like those of immunoglobulin, are unusual in that the complete gene is put together only during T-cell development by recombining different gene fragments (see Figs 10 and 12). Thus, T and B cells break the dogma that all cells carry identical genomic DNA sequences.

Chemokine ligands (CCLs) and their receptors (CCR) A large related family of genes coding for soluble messengers, and their receptors (see Fig. 23), which have a key role in directing the localization and migration of all immune cells. There are two main clusters of chemokine genes, coding for two different, although related, families, and one major cluster of chemokine receptor genes. A genomic deletion (absence of sequence) is present in about 1% of white Caucasians, which results in a complete absence of the CCR5 receptor. Remarkably, this deletion confers almost complete protection against HIV infection. The absence of CCR5, however, predisposes to another human pathogen, African West Nile virus, perhaps accounting for the absence of this deletion in African populations.

Cytokines act as messengers between one immune cell and another, binding to specific target receptors, and hence orchestrating the complex series of events that constitute an immune response (see Figs 23 and 24). There are several families of structurally related cytokines (only one example is shown, for simplicity). Defects in the **IL-17 receptor** predispose to serious mucocutaneous fungal infection, while mutant forms of the IL-12 and **IFNγ receptor** increase the risk of developing tuberculosis. Defects in the genes coding for components of the cytokine signalling pathways (e.g. the DNA-binding protein **STAT3**) can lead to complex and often life-threatening failures in the proper regulation of immune responses.

CD28 family of cell surface receptors are found especially on T cells, where they interact principally with members of the B7 family of ligands. These molecules have a critical role in regulating the magnitude and termination of immune response. A small group of volunteers were injected with a monoclonal antibody specific for CD28, as part of a trial for a potential therapeutic for autoimmune disease. Instead, the injection resulted in massive uncontrolled inflammatory response, almost killing some of the volunteers – a warning of the complexity of the immune system, and the potential dangers of tampering with it!

Mutations in the ***autoimmune regulator gene (AIRE)***, which regulates protein expression in the thymus, and in the **FAS and FAS ligand** receptors which regulate apoptosis can lead to a breakdown of self-tolerance (see Fig. 22), and consequent autoimmune disease (see Fig. 38).

Type I interferons A family of antiviral proteins that also have powerful immunomodulatory activities (see Fig. 2). Several genetic defects in the signalling machinery that transmits the interferon signal have been linked to increased susceptibility to several viruses (one such gene, *UNC93B*, is linked to herpes simplex encephalitis), and this is turn may lead to serious asthma. Remarkably, the human genome contains genes for 13 type I interferons, all of which bind to the same receptor. The biological significance of this remains totally mysterious, but may be related to the need to switch on interferon production in so many different cell types, and under so many different situations.

Mutations that reduce the activity of the enzyme NAPDH oxidase result in a reduced ability of phagocytes to kill bacteria, and were one of the first mutations shown to lead to a specific deficiency of innate immunity, chronic granulomatous disease (see Fig. 33). Mutations in an **iron transporting protein, NRAMP,** also impair innate immunity and increase the risk of tuberculosis and leprosy. An interesting recent discovery is that immunodeficient individuals who carry a mutation in the DNA binding protein IRF8 have a complete absence of monocytes and dendritic cells.

Toll-like receptors The prototype pathogen recogntion receptors of innate immunity (see Fig. 5). The human genome contains 10 functional TLRs recognizing a wide range of viral and bacterial components. A genetic defect in TLR5, which recognizes a major component of bacterial flagellae, predisposes to Legionnaires' disease.

Immunoglobulins The antigen-specific receptor on B cells is discussed in detail in Fig 14. Like T-cell receptors, immunoglobulin chains are put together by rearranging genomic fragments during lymphocyte development (for details see Fig. 14). A remarkable achievement of genetic engineering has been to introduce the whole genomic sequence coding for human light and heavy chains into a mouse. This allows production of completely 'human' antibodies, which can be used for therapeutic purposes without the danger of being recognized as foreign, using all the techniques of classic mouse immunology.

Major histocompatibility complex An enormous complex of genes (many of unknown function) stretching over 3.6 megabases on chromosome 6, which includes the classic class I and II major histocompatibility molecules that direct peptide presentation to the T cell (see Fig. 11). These genes are the most polymorphic known, with hundreds of different alleles of some chains already described. These differences have received enormous attention, partly because they determine the strength with which grafts between different individuals are rejected, but also because particular variants are associated with many infectious, autoimmune and allergic diseases.

X-linked immunodeficiencies (see Fig. 33). The X chromosome is the only one that is found 'unpaired' in males, as males have a Y chromosome in place of a second X chromosome. For this reason, recessive mutations on X chromosomes can behave as dominant in males, giving rise to the so-called sex-linked diseases. Several X-linked immunological diseases have been described. Two examples are shown in the figure. A defect in the **IL-2 receptor gamma chain**, a receptor required for lymphocyte development, gives rise to severe combined immunodeficiency syndrome, in which all lymphocyte development is blocked at an early stage. This disease is one of the first to have been treated successfully by the new gene therapy technologies (see Fig. 33). In contrast, a defect in **CD40** ligand, a receptor on the surface of B cells, gives rise to a more subtle immunodeficiency, hyper IgM syndrome, in which B cells cannot receive the correct signals from T cells and are therefore arrested at the IgM production stage, rather than switching to IgG as the immune response progresses.

Self-assessment questions

Below you will find four sets of typical exam essay questions, based on chapters in this book. Make short notes for an answer and then compare them with the specimen notes on the following pages. Remember – there is no perfect essay: what examiners look for is an understanding of the subject. A few errors or omissions will not pull you down as much as unstructured verbiage, repetition and, above all, plagiarism. Sometimes the full answer to the question is not known; here you may have to give an opinion, but it should be clearly argued.

Paper 1 (based on Figures 1–9)

1 *What are the main differences between innate and adaptive immunity?*
2 *The immune system exists to interact with pathogenic microorganisms. Where exactly is the interface between pathogen and host?*
3 *What role(s) does complement have in immunity?*
4 *How do phagocytic cells recognize foreign microorganisms?*
5 *Is inflammation a good or a bad thing?*

Paper 2 (based on Figures 10–25)

1 *What properties distinguish lymphocytes from phagocytes?*
2 *How do T cells differ from B cells?*
3 *What are the main steps in mounting an antibody response?*
4 *How does the structure of the antibody molecule relate to its function?*

5 *How does the major histocompatibility complex (MHC) contribute to immune responses?*
6 *What do the terms 'primary' and 'secondary' lymphoid organs mean?*
7 *What do the various cytokines have in common?*
8 *With what other body systems does the immune system interact?*

Paper 3 (based on Figures 26–39)

1 *The immune system handles intracellular and extracellular microorganisms differently. Discuss.*
2 *What can an infectious microorganism do to avoid elimination by the immune system?*
3 *When is an immune response a bad thing?*
4 *Distinguish between autoimmunity and autoimmune disease.*
5 *Why are kidney grafts rejected and what can be done about it?*

Paper 4 (based on Figures 40–47)

1 *Name and describe two infectious diseases that cause immunosuppression.*
2 *Why are some vaccines more effective than others?*
3 *How can a drug influence the immune system?*
4 *Immunology and the kidney. Discuss.*
5 *Name four laboratory tests used to evaluate immune status.*

Immunology at a Glance, Tenth Edition. J.H.L. Playfair and B.M. Chain. © 2013 John Wiley & Sons, Ltd. Published 2013 by John Wiley & Sons, Ltd.

Answers

Your answer should include discussion of at least some of the following topics.

Paper 1

1 Innate: invertebrates and vertebrates; importance of phagocytes; recognition of pathogen surface patterns. Adaptive: vertebrates only; based on lymphocytes; high receptor diversity, thus specificity; memory.

2 Innate: pathogen-associated molecular patterns (PAMP) and pattern-recognizing receptors (PRR). Adaptive: B- and T-lymphocyte receptors and microbial molecules.

3 Promotes phagocytosis, promotes inflammation, lyses some bacteria; all enhanced by antibody.

4 By their own PRRs; also via receptors for microorganism-bound antibody and/or complement.

5 Good in allowing increased supply of blood and its contents (cells, molecules) to the site; bad in causing pain, tissue damage.

Paper 2

1 Lymphocytes recirculate; rearrange their receptor genes, thus highly specific for antigen; proliferate into clones; can survive as memory cells. Phagocytes less specific; react faster; no memory.

2 T cells carry TCR (α/β or γ/δ); secrete cytokines (TH), kill target cells (CTL). B cells carry surface immunogloblin, T cells predominate in blood.

3 Antigen uptake and processing in B cells; antigen uptake and processing in antigen-presenting cells (APCs); presentation by APCs to T cells; increased antibody synthesis and secretion by B cells; class switching; regulation. Note: some antigens do not require the T-cell stage.

4 Fab variable, binds antigen, highly discriminatory. Fc mediates function, binding to phagocytes, complement, mast cells; class differences; switching.

5 T cells only recognize antigen when small peptides bind to major histocompatibility complex (MHC) on either B cells and macrophages (MHC II) or target (e.g. virus-infected) cells (MHC I). MHC essentially unique to individual, so a problem in transplantation. Some diseases, especially autoimmune, MHC linked.

6 Primary: essential to lymphocyte development; removal blocks, e.g. thymus T cells. Secondary: site of recirculation and responses, e.g. lymph nodes.

7 They are low molecular weight proteins, secreted by one cell to stimulate or inhibit others. Rather elastic term conventionally restricted to immune and haemopoietic system; many made by T cells or macrophages.

8 The endocrine system: effect of hormones on immunity; endocrine organs frequently target of autoimmunity. The central nervous system; shared mediators; psychological effects on disease susceptibility immunological?

Paper 3

1 Extracellular organisms, in the blood or tissue spaces, should be recognized by the receptors on phagocytes, B cells, and molecules such as antibody and complement. However, these cannot penetrate inside cells to 'see' their contents. This is where T cells (and the MHC) come in. As a rough generalization, phagocytes, antibody and complement deal with extracellular infections, T cells with intracellular ones.

2 They can suppress immunity (staphylococci versus phagocytes, HIV versus T cells), confuse it (antigenic variation), hide from it (intracellular habitat).

3 When it is an over-reaction (allergy, complex-mediated inflammation, granuloma) or directed against 'self' antigens (autoimmunity).

4 Autoimmunity requires the demonstration of antibody or T cells that react to 'self'; autoimmune disease requires that they cause symptoms.

5 Because they carry 'non-self' MHC and therefore stimulate host T cells, leading to both antibody and cytotoxic responses. Tissue typing and matching and immunosuppression are the main counter-strategies.

Paper 4

1 HIV infection is the worst one; infects CD4 T cells, macrophages, suppresses cell-mediated immunity. Malaria suppresses antibody responses. Also measles, TB, Epstein–Barr virus (EBV) infection, trypanosomiasis.

2 Living vaccines usually better than dead: right site, longer persistence. Vaccine may induce wrong type of immunity. Immunity may not be effective (e.g. antigenic variation). Animal reservoirs.

3 Immunosuppression (steroids, ciclosporin). Hypersensitivity – especially penicillin. Immunostimulation (e.g. by cytokines) still experimental.

4 Glomerulonephritis often type III hypersensitivity (complex mediated), more rarely autoimmune (Goodpasture's; also lung). Kidney is the most common organ transplanted; importance of MHC. May be affected in vasculitis, myeloma, amyloid.

5 Blood count (lymphocytes, T, B, NK); serum immunoglobulins, complement; skin tests (immediate: allergy; delayed, e.g. Mantoux); immunofluoresence for autoantibodies in blood or tissue sections.

Appendix I

Comparative sizes

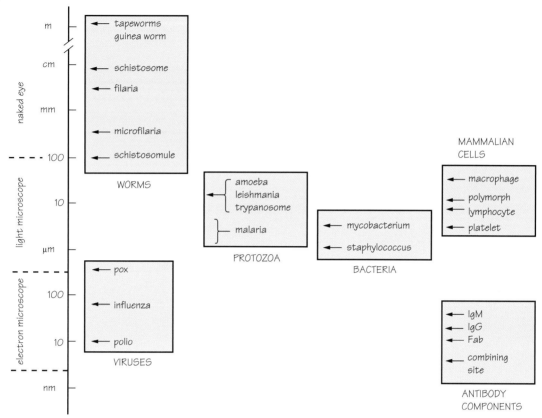

Comparative molecular weights

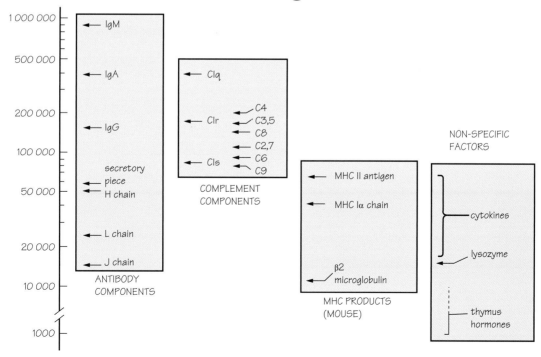

Appendix II

Landmarks in the history of immunology

1798	Jenner: vaccination against smallpox; the beginning of immunology
1881–5	Pasteur: attenuated vaccines (cholera, anthrax, rabies)
1882	Metchnikoff: phagocytosis (in starfish)
1888	Roux, Yersin: diphtheria antitoxin (antibody)
1890	Von Behring: passive protection (tetanus) by antibody
1891	Koch: delayed hypersensitivity (tuberculosis)
1893	Buchner: heat-labile serum factor (complement)
1896	Widal: diagnosis by antibody (typhoid)
1897	Ehrlich: 'side chain' (receptor) theory
1900	Landsteiner: ABO groups in blood transfusion
1902	Portier and Richet: hypersensitivity
1903	Arthus: local anaphylaxis
1906	Von Pirquet: allergy
1910	Dale: histamine
1917–	Landsteiner: haptens, carriers and antibody specificity
1922	Fleming: lysozyme
1924	Glenny: adjuvants
1936	Gorer: transplantation antigens
1938	Tiselius and Kabat: antibodies as gamma-globulins
1943	Chase: transfer of delayed hypersensitivity by cells
1944–	Medawar: skin graft rejection as an immune response
1945	Coombs: antiglobulin test for red-cell autoantibody
1947	Owen: tolerance in cattle twins
1952	Bruton: agammaglobulinaemia
1953	Billingham, Brent and Medawar: neonatal induction of tolerance
1956	Glick: bursa dependence of antibody response
1956	Roitt and Doniach: autoantibodies in thyroid disease
1957	Isaacs and Lindenman: interferon
1958	Gell and Coombs: classification of hypersensitivities
1959	Porter, Edelman: enzyme cleavage of antibody molecule
1959	Gowans: lymphocyte recirculation
1959	Burnet: clonal selection theory

1960	Nowell: lymphocyte transformation (PHA)
1961–2	Miller, Good: thymus dependence of immune responses
1965	DiGeorge: thymus deficiency
1966	David, Bloom and Bennett: macrophage activation by cytokines
1966–7	Claman; Davies; Mitchison: cooperation of T and B cells
1968	Dausset: HLA
1969	McDevitt: immune response genes
1971	Gershon: suppression by T cells
1972	Borel: ciclosporin
1973	Steinmann: dendritic cells
1974	Jerne: network theory of immune regulation
1975	Unanue: antigen processing for class II MHC
1975	Zinkernagel and Doherty; Bevan, Shevach: dual recognition by T cells
1975	Köhler and Milstein: monoclonal antibodies from hybridomas
1976	Tonegawa: immunoglobulin gene rearrangement
1980	Smallpox eradicated
1981	AIDS recognized
1982	First recombinant subunit vaccine for hepatitis B
1984–	Marrack, Davis, Hedrick: T-cell receptor structure and genetics
1986–	Townsend, Braciale: antigen processing for class I MHC
1986–	Coffman and Mosmann: T^{H1} and T^{H2} subsets
1987	Bjorkman: structure of MHC class I molecule
1990	Wolff, Tang: DNA immunization
1993	Feldmann, Maini: anti-TNFα therapy for RA
1996	Wilson, Wiley: T-cell receptor/MHC co-crystal
1996–8	Janeway, Hoffman and Beutler: pattern recognition and Toll-like receptors
2007	Human papillomavirus vaccine: the first successful vaccine against cancer

Some unsolved problems

AIDS Why do so many T cells die? Will a vaccine ever succeed?

Autoimmunity Can we cure it ? Can T^{REG} help? What are the genetic predispositions involved?

Cancer How much can immunology help?

Cytokines (interleukins, interferons, growth factors). Why so much overlap in function?

HLA and disease How and why are they associated?

Human organ grafting What are the critical antigens and will specific tolerance be possible?

Immunodeficiency Will gene therapy be the cure?

Psychoneuroimmunology Fact or fad?

Systems biology Can we simplify the complexity of the immune system mathematically?

T cells How do regulatory T cells work?

Tolerance How important is the thymus? How do T^{REG} really work?

Vaccination Will the parasite diseases succumb? How does the 'naked DNA' vaccine work? How to combat bioterrorism?

Appendix III

CD classification

CD (cluster of differentiation) numbers are used to identify cell-surface antigens that can be distinguished by monoclonal antibodies. Some of these (e.g. CD25, CD35, CD71) are clear-cut functional molecules, and several (e.g. CD3, CD4, CD8) are also widely used as markers of particular cell types. The table below shows some of the CDs identified so far, which contain many of the key functional molecules on lymphocytes and myeloid cells. In many cases, the original 'common' name of the molecule is still widely used. The assignment of new CDs is carried out by the Human Cell Differentiation Molecules organization. A full list of all 363 CDs assigned to date can be found at their website: www.hcdm.org

CD number	Function	Distribution
1a–c	Non-peptide antigen presentation	T, B, DC
2	Costimulation	T
3	Antigen-specific T-cell activation	T
4	T-cell costimulation	T, M, DC
5	Costimulation	T, some B
6	Adhesion/costimulation	T, some B
7	T–T and T–B interaction	T
8	Costimulation	T
9	Costimulation/adhesion/activation	T, B, P, E
10	Endopeptidase	B, G, other
11a–c	Adhesion (integrin α chains)	T, B, M, DC, G
12	Not known	T
13	Aminopeptidase N	M, DC, G, E
14	LPS receptor	M
15	Adhesion (Lewis X)	M, G
16	Low-affinity IgG receptor	M
17	Not known	Widespread
18	Adhesion (integrin β2 chain)	B, T, M, G
19	Costimulation	B
20	Costimulation	B
21	Complement receptor	B
22	Adhesion/costimulation	B
23	Low-affinity IgE receptor	B
24	Adhesion, apoptosis	B, G
25	IL-2 receptor chain	T
26	Dipeptidyl peptidase	E
27	Costimulation	T, B
28	Costimulation	T
29	Adhesion (integrin β1)	Widespread
30	Costimulation	B
31	Adhesion	M, G, E
32	Low-affinity IgG receptor	M, G, P
33	Adhesion	M, G
34	Adhesion	E
35	Complement receptor	M, G
36	Scavenger receptor	M, P
37	Costimulation, signal transduction	T, B
38	ADP-ribosyl cyclase	T, B
39	Not known	B, ??
40	Costimulation	B, M, DC
41	Adhesion (integrin)	P
42a–d	Adhesion	T, P
43	Adhesion/anti-adhesion	T, B, M, DC, G
44	Adhesion/costimulation	T, B, M, DC, G
45, 45RA, B, C, O	Costimulation, T-cell memory marker	Widespread
46	Complement regulator	Widespread
47	Adhesion	Widespread
48	Adhesion	Widespread

CD number	Function	Distribution
49a–f	Adhesion (integrin α1–6 chains)	Widespread
50	Adhesion (ICAM)	B, T, M, DC, G
51	Adhesion (integrin α chain)	P, E
52	Not known	T, B, M
53	Costimulation	T, B, M, G
54	Adhesion (ICAM)	Widespread
55	Complement regulation	Widespread
56	Adhesion	NK
57	Adhesion	NK, ??
58	Costimulation	Widespread
59	Complement regulation	Widespread
60a–c	Costimulation	P, E
61	Adhesion (integrin β3)	P, E
62E, 62L, 62P	Adhesion, homing	Widespread
63	Tetraspan integrin receptor	M, G, P, E
64	High-affinity IgG receptor	M
65	Adhesion	M, G
66a–f	Costimulation, adhesion	G
67	Alternative name for CD66b	G
68	Lysosomal receptor	M
69	Costimulation, activation	T, M, G, P
70	Costimulation	B
71	Transferrin receptor	B, T
72	CD5 ligand	B
73	Ecto-5′-nucleotidase	B
74	Antigen processing (invariant chain)	T, B, M, DC
75s	Lactosamines, adhesion	B, T
76	Merged with CD75s	B
77	Apoptosis	B
78	Not assigned	
79a,b	Antigen-specific activation	B
80	Costimulation	B, DC
81	Costimulation	T, B
82	Costimulation	T, B, M, G
83	Antigen presentation	B, DC
84	Antigen presentation	B, M
85	Inhibitory signalling receptors recognizing MHC	T, B, DC, NK
86	Costimulation	B, M, DC
87	Urokinase plasminogen activator receptor	Widespread
88	Complement receptor	M, G
89	Fcα receptor	M, G
90	Haemopoiesis (Thy 1)	T, B, E
91	α2-Macroglobulin receptor	M
92	Lipid transport and metabolism	T, B, M, G
93	C1q receptor, removal of apoptotic cells	M, G, E

CD number	Function	Distribution
94	NK inhibitory receptor	NK
95	Apoptosis	T, B, E
96	Adhesion	T, NK
97	Adhesion	T, B, M, G
98	Amino acid transport, adhesion, cell activation	Widespread
99	Apoptosis	T, B, P, E
100	Costimulation	Widespread
101	Costimulation	M
102	Adhesion (ICAM)	??
103	Adhesion (integrin)	T, B
104	Adhesion (integrin)	T, B, E
105	TGF-coreceptor	E
106	Adhesion	E
107a, b	Not known (LAMP)	B, E
108	Not known	Widespread
109	Not known	T, E
110	Platelet production (TPO receptor)	P
111	Chemokine receptor	M
112	Chemokine receptor	M
113	Not assigned	
114	Haemopoiesis	G, P
115	M-CSF receptor	B, M
116	GM-CSF receptor	M, G
117	Haemopoiesis	S
118	Not assigned	
119	IFNγ receptor	Widespread
120a, b	TNF-α receptor	Widespread
121a, b	IL-1 receptor	Widespread
122	IL-2, IL-15 receptor	T, B
123	IL-3 receptor	Widespread
124	IL-4/IL-13 receptor	T, B
125	IL-5 receptor	B
126	IL-6 receptor	Widespread
127	IL-7 receptor	T
128	Chemokine receptor	M, G
130	IL-6, IL-11, and multiple other cytokine receptors	E
131	IL-3, IL-5, GM-CSF receptor	Widespread
132	IL-2, IL-4, IL-7, IL-9, L-15 receptor	T, B
133	Haemopoiesis (?)	Stem cells
134	Adhesion/costimulation	T
135	Haemopoiesis	Immature cells only
136	Differentiation	Immature cells only

CD number	Function	Distribution
137	Costimulation	T
138	Adhesion	T, B
139	Not known	Widespread
140	PDGF receptor	E
141	Blood clotting	E
142	Blood clotting	E
143	Angiotensin-converting enzyme	E
144	Adhesion	E
145	Not known	E
146	Adhesion (?)	B, E
147	Adhesion (?)	Widespread
148	Activation (?)	Widespread
149	Reclassified as 47	
150	Costimulation	T, B
151	Adhesion	Widespread
152	Costimulation	T, B
153	Costimulation	T, B
154	Costimulation	T, B
155	Not known (poliovirus receptor)	T, E
156	Metalloproteinase	M, G
157	ADP-ribosyl cyclase	M, G
158a, b	NK inhibitory receptor	NK
159	NK inhibitory receptor	NK
160	Costimulation (?)	T, NK
161	NK inhibitory receptor	NK
162	Adhesion	Not known
163	Not known	Not known
164	Adhesion	Widespread
165	Adhesion	T, P
166	Adhesion	T, B, E
206	Mannose receptor	M
212	IL-2 receptor subunit	T, various
230	Prion protein	Neurones
234	Duffy antigen	RBC
281–289	TLR innate immune recognition	Widespread
324–325	Cadherin, adhesion	Epithelium
340	Her2Neu, growth receptor	Epithelium
361	S1P receptor 1, migration	Endothelium

The distribution shows the major expression on the following cell types only: B, B cells; DC, dendritic cells; E, endothelium; G, granulocyte; M, monocyte/macrophage; NK, natural killer cells; P, platelets; PDGF, platelet-derived growth factor; LAMP, Lysosome-associated membrane protein, RBC, red blood cells; T, T cells; TPO, thrombopoetin receptor, ??, distribution still doubtful.

Index

Numbers indicate page number. Numbers in **bold** indicate principal references.

Keep up with critical fields

Would you like to receive up-to-date information on our books, journals and databases in the areas that interest you, direct to your mailbox?

Join the **Wiley e-mail service** - a convenient way to receive updates and exclusive discount offers on products from us.

Simply visit **www.wiley.com/email** and register online

We won't bombard you with emails and we'll only email you with information that's relevant to you. We will ALWAYS respect your e-mail privacy and NEVER sell, rent, or exchange your e-mail address to any outside company. Full details on our privacy policy can be found online.

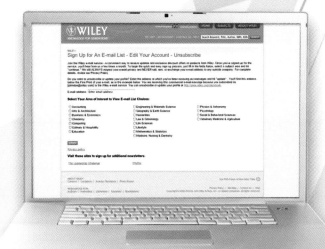

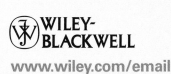

WILEY-BLACKWELL

www.wiley.com/email

17841

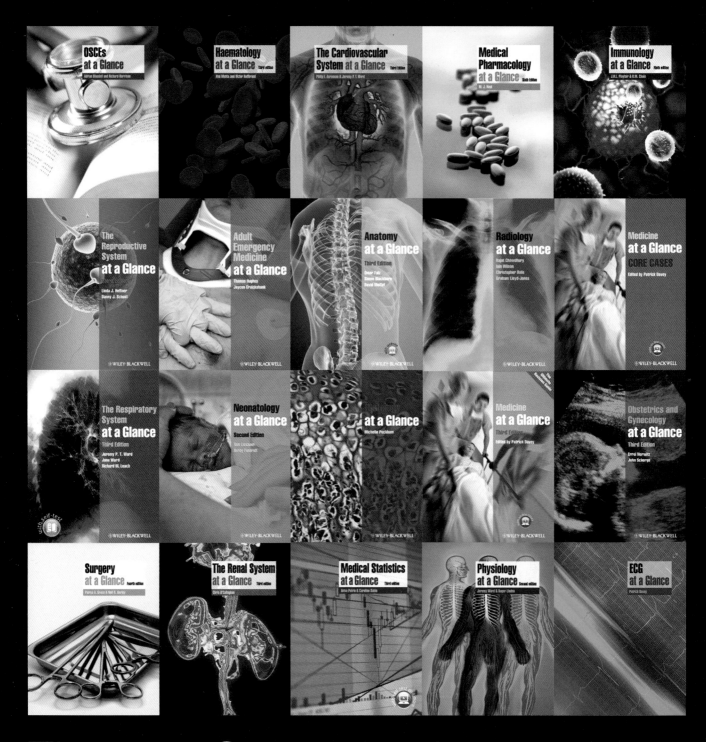

The at a Glance series

Popular double-page spread format • Coverage of core knowledge
Full-colour throughout • Self-assessment to test your knowledge • Expert authors

www.wileymedicaleducation.com

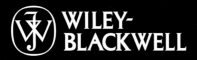

WILEY-BLACKWELL